COMPLETE GUIDE TO GOOD SEX

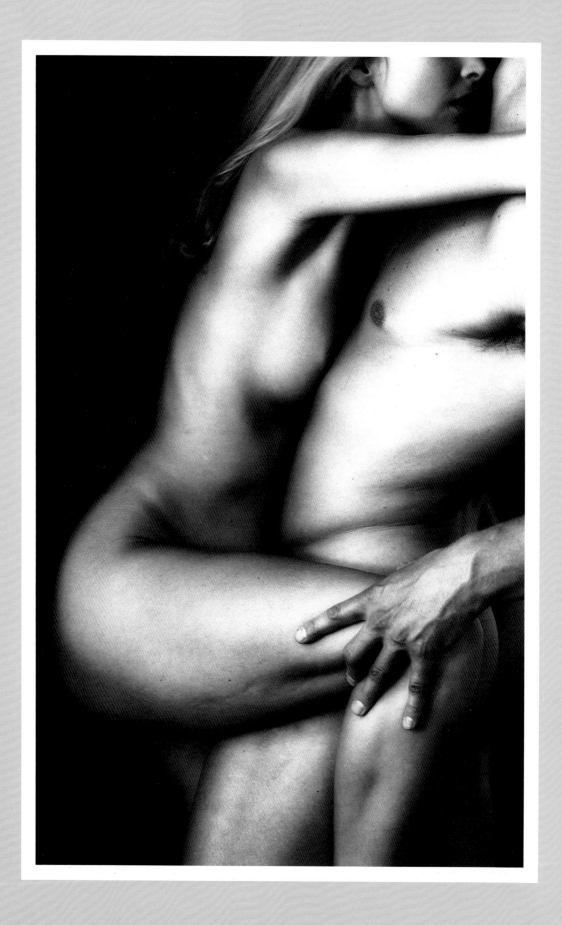

a consultation with **DR VERNON COLEMAN**

COMPLETE GUIDE
TO GOOD SEX

HAMLYN

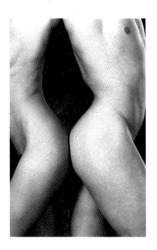

NOTE

THIS BOOK IS NOT INTENDED AS AN ALTERNATIVE TO PERSONAL,
PROFESSIONAL MEDICAL ADVICE. THE READER SHOULD CONSULT
A PHYSICIAN IN ALL MATTERS RELATING TO HEALTH AND
PARTICULARLY IN RESPECT OF ANY SYMPTOMS WHICH MAY REQUIRE
DIAGNOSIS OR MEDICAL ATTENTION. WHILE THE ADVICE AND
INFORMATION ARE BELIEVED TO BE ACCURATE AND TRUE AT THE TIME
OF GOING TO PRESS NEITHER THE AUTHOR NOR THE PUBLISHER CAN
ACCEPT ANY LEGAL RESPONSIBILITY OR LIABILITY FOR ANY ERRORS
OR OMISSIONS THAT MAY BE MADE.

FIRST PUBLISHED IN GREAT BRITAIN 1993
BY HAMLYN, AN IMPRINT OF REED CONSUMER BOOKS LIMITED,
MICHELIN HOUSE, 81 FULHAM ROAD, LONDON SW3 6RB
AND AUCKLAND, MELBOURNE, SINGAPORE AND TORONTO

COPYRIGHT © VERNON COLEMAN 1993
DESIGN AND ILLUSTRATIONS © REED INTERNATIONAL BOOKS LIMITED 1993

ISBN 0 600 57576 4

A CIP RECORD FOR THIS BOOK IS AVAILABLE AT THE BRITISH LIBRARY

PRINTED IN ITALY

CONTENTS

CHAPTER ONE

Him And Her

Many of the sexual problems that cause anxiety and frustration and that damage relationships arise through simple ignorance. To make a good lover you need to know as much as possible about the sexual equipment of your partner – and how it works! If you are confident that you know everything there is to know about the opposite sex then you can skip much of this chapter. But if you want to know what really happens during an orgasm read on...

HIM

The male sexual equipment is stored outside the body and is, therefore, highly visible to any observer. It consists of a penis and a scrotum (or sack) which holds the two testicles. Male sexual equipment has two simple jobs to do: production and distribution.

The production task involves the preparation of a large quantity of good quality sperm. Each individual sperm is very small and in order to ensure that there is a fighting chance that an egg will be fertilized, it is essential that a huge number of sperm are made. Quality and quantity are the two criteria by which the production department is judged. Production of sperm is carried out in the two testicles which are stored outside the body, so that the local temperature doesn't rise too much. The sperm production department won't work properly if the temperature rises too high.

Although no one notices if the production department fails to produce good quantities of well-made sperm, everyone notices if the distribution department doesn't do its job properly.

The task of the distribution department is to deposit as many as possible of those sperm close to a woman's womb, so that they have a decent chance of reaching and fertilizing an egg. It is

the distribution aspect of the male function that attracts most interest and is responsible for most sexual problems.

The simple problem that the distribution department has to overcome is the fact that the egg waiting to be fertilized is hidden quite deep inside the woman's body. If the sperm were left at the entrance to the vagina they would never get there in time. They would die, exhausted and frustrated, long before they reached their target. To solve the problem the male body uses the penis to deposit the sperm as close as possible to the target – the womb.

In its normal state the male penis is quite limp and flaccid and rather small. It is perfectly adequate for passing urine but as a tool for entering the female vagina it lacks one vital quality: rigidity. Try threading a needle with a dangling end of cotton and you'll soon understand what I mean.

Extraordinary as it may seem, there is some available evidence to suggest that many thousands of years ago the male penis may have had a bone in it to make penetration much easier. In France just thirty or so years ago doctors produced X ray evidence of a male with a small bone in his penis. However, a bone fixed to the pelvis wouldn't really be practical.

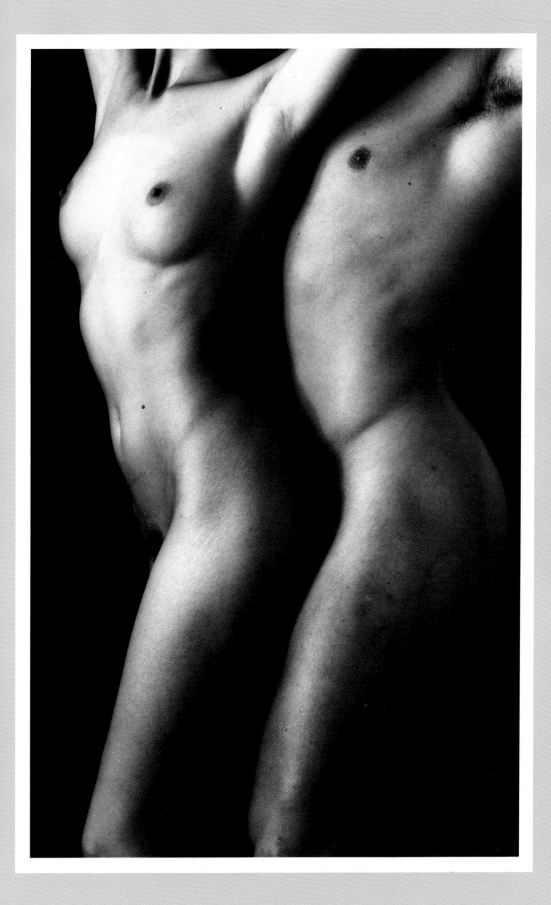

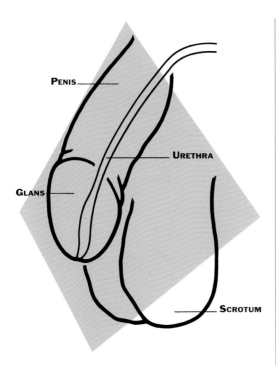

PENIS

URETHRA

GLANS

SCROTUM

would be completely impossible in anything other than a few unusual sexual positions. If the penis pointed upwards, then every man would be forever urinating up towards the ceiling. And trousers would have to be redesigned!

So, the penis behaves quite differently when performing its two very separate functions. When acting as a conduit for urine the penis remains limp. But when being used as a distribution aid for sperm it becomes larger and more erect so that it can deposit sperm safely inside the vagina.

THE ANATOMY OF THE PENIS

All penises have much the same general structure (whatever their sizes). At birth the male penis consists of two clearly defined parts: the shaft and the more sensitive glans. The glans is partly or completely covered by the foreskin, a loose extension of the skin which covers the rest of the penis. Underneath the penis a fairly thin fold of skin – the frenulum – holds the glans to the shaft of the penis. If the frenulum is unusually short it will prevent the penis from becoming properly erect and will lead to premature ejaculation. In well over ninety per cent of male babies the foreskin is so tight that it cannot be drawn back from the glans, but by the time a boy reaches puberty his foreskin will have usually become much looser. When male hormones circulate at puberty the glans pushes out through the foreskin. A number

God or nature long ago decided to economize with male architecture, and so in addition to serving its vital role as a male sexual organ, the penis also has to function as a discharge tube for urine; both semen and urine come out through the same opening in the centre of the glans at the end of the penis. A valve ensures that the penis is only used to urinate when it is limp – a man cannot urinate when he has an erection.

If the penis had a bone in it, which way would it point? If it pointed downwards, penetration

Circumsized penis

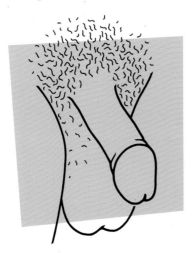

Uncircumsized penis

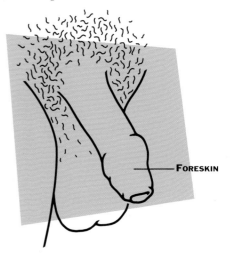

FORESKIN

of small glands on the inner surface of the double fold, produced by the foreskin, produce a type of lubricating grease which helps to protect the extremely sensitive glans.

For a variety of reasons, usually health or religious, the foreskin is sometimes removed during an operation known as circumcision, but it is important to remember that this apparently useless piece of skin does exist for a purpose. Its job is to protect the glans from irritation. In men who have no foreskin, the urethral opening often gets gradually smaller and smaller as a result of irritation, inflammation and hardening of the unprotected glans. There is, in addition, some evidence that another unwelcome effect of circircumcision is that the glans will become slightly less sensitive.

THE AVERAGE SIZE OF AN AVERAGE MALE PENIS – WHEN ERECT

The male penis is born with the necessary physiological equipment to become erect. And the maximum erect size of a penis grows as its owner grows – though not necessarily in proportion to the eventual overall size of the individual. The height and weight of the owner have little influence on the size of a penis. It is a myth that you can tell the size of a man's penis by looking at his overall height or the size of his nose or feet.

At birth the average erect penis is little more than one inch (2.5 cms) long. By the time a boy reaches the age of twelve his erect penis will probably be around two inches (5 cms) long. And then things usually start to improve fairly dramatically. By the age of fifteen the average erect penis is around five inches (12.5 cms) long and by full adulthood the average erect penis is around six and a half inches (nearly 17 cms) long and three and a half inches (9 cms) in circumference. The size of an adult penis tends to increase slightly with age. This is one of the very few physical benefits for men associated with ageing and the length of a fairly ordinary, average-sized sort of penis can increase by as much as an inch

throughout its owner's entire adult lifetime.

The size of the average penis seems to have become slightly bigger over the last century or so. Medical surveys carried out in the late nineteenth century showed that the length of the average penis ranged between three inches and four and a half inches (between 7.5 cms and 11.5 cms) in length, so there seems to have been a healthy increase in the last hundred years or so. The majority of men are remarkably close to this average size. Genuine under or over-development is relatively rare and is usually accompanied by other signs of poor development: there is, in fact, far more variation in the size of female breasts than there is in the size of male penises.

FROM LIMP TO FIRM

There is a considerable change in the size of a penis when it becomes erect and penis size tends to even out rather a lot during the process of erection. The length, width and general size of a penis at rest gives absolutely no indication of its potential size when aroused. In some men the main effect of erection is to increase the length of the penis. In others it is to increase the width. In some men erection has a relatively slight effect on the size of the penis. A penis which is small when limp may, when erect, become larger than a penis which promised much when limp.

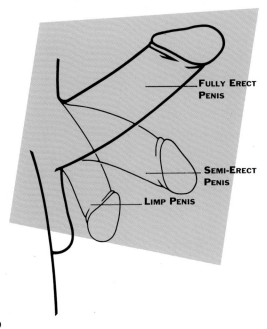

FULLY ERECT PENIS

SEMI-ERECT PENIS

LIMP PENIS

> **TO MEASURE A PENIS GENTLY GRASP THE END OF THE ERECT PENIS BETWEEN THUMB AND FIRST FINGER AND LIE IT ALONG A RULER WHICH HAS ONE END PUSHED FIRMLY AGAINST THE MALE PUBIC BONE. MEASURE TO THE TIP OF THE GLANS NOT TO THE END OF A STRETCHED FORESKIN.**

HOW LONG IS TOO SMALL?

Men worry a great deal about the size of their penis, and whatever Freud may say, true penis envy is more common among men than among women. Men worry about the size of their penises about as much as women worry about the size of their breasts (which is very often). This obsession with size is not confined to homo sapiens. Among some monkeys the one with the largest penis is automatically made the 'boss' while the size of a baboon's penis plays a vital part in his acceptance (or otherwise) by the local female population.

Unfortunately many young boys often feel under-endowed when they look around in the school showers. What they do not realize is that boys of a similar age may have reached puberty much earlier and their organs may, therefore, have started to get larger sooner. Adult men also suffer the same fears. What they fail to realize is that each man's view of his own penis is short-ened by an optical illusion when he looks down on it. If two men face one another naked both will almost always think that the other has a con-siderably larger penis. Some comfort can usually be obtained by looking into a mirror where a more accurate view can be obtained.

Most of these fears are unfounded anyway. There is no correlation between the size of a man's penis and his ability to satisfy a woman in bed. When women do find large penises more exciting it is usually because they look more

exciting rather than because they provide more sexual satisfaction. Some women like to admire large penises in the same way that some men like to admire large breasts. The admiration is largely artistic rather than functional.

CAN A PENIS BE TOO BIG?

Occasionally a man may worry that his penis is too big. And some women worry that if a man has too large a penis it may hurt them during sex. Theoretically it *is* possible that an unusually large penis could hurt a woman, but the risk is fairly small since the female vagina can expand and adapt itself to cope with a baby's head (which is rather larger than any penis ever recorded). The only real hazard is that if a penis is exceptionally long it could deposit sperm in the vaginal cul-de-sac behind the cervix. This would make it difficult for sperm to get into the womb and so reduce the chances of the woman getting preg-nant. In addition, a very long penis could cause pain by lifting the uterus upwards. To balance this risk there is the fact that a penis long enough to touch the cervix during love-making may trig-ger an orgasm as it does so. The only other point worth making about extra large penises is that a man with an unusually large organ will need to have a very strong erection. A man with an exceptionally large organ will probably not be able to get away with a half-hearted erection because he will have difficulty in pushing his member between the woman's labia minora (the inner lips of the vagina) into the vagina.

WIDTH AND LENGTH

The thickness of a penis has far more effect than the length of a penis on a woman's chance of reaching an orgasm during vaginal sex. The unstretched vagina is usually around four to five inches (10 to 12.5 cms) long, so the average penis is longer than is necessary to reach the cervix. It is the thickness of the penis which decides how much the labia minora will be moved during intercourse and it is this move-ment which stimulates the clitoris and produces the female orgasm. Although many women may find a long, slender penis attractive to look at, the fact is that a short, fat penis is more likely to provide sexual satisfaction.

SEMEN –
WHAT IT CONTAINS

Semen is whitish, with a yellowish tinge, and an average ejaculate contains around 5 mls (about a teaspoonful). Men who want to obtain a more copious ejaculate can do so by masturbating nearly but not quite to orgasm an hour or so before sex. This increases the amount of prostatic secretion – and therefore the quantity of semen.

The primary constituent of semen – the fluid produced when a man ejaculates – is sperm (although there are no spermatozoa in semen until a teenager reaches the age of about seventeen). Men produce sperm all the time and the seminal vesicles or storage sacs inside their testicles are full of it. On an average sort of day a healthy man will produce around 90 million sperm – enough to populate North America in half a week or the whole of northern Europe in one week. Sperm production is fast and after having sex a normal, healthy man's sperm storage sacs will be full again in just two or three days. If a man doesn't have sex regularly then his sperm producing skills will diminish as will his body's production of testosterone (the male hormone), and therefore, so will his sexual drive.

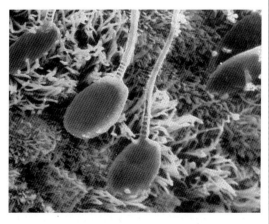

A healthy man produces approximately 90 million sperm evey day

As well as sperm, semen contains many different ingredients which together produce its well-known horse chestnut pollen smell and salty taste. There are proteins, sugar, vitamin C and secretions from the prostate gland which stimulate the production of sperm. Semen is so rich in nutrients that in some African tribes it is collected during initiation ceremonies and afterwards used as a remedy for a wide variety of ailments. In many primitive societies women regard semen as a precious foodstuff, and today numerous scientists claim that semen contains ingredients which can improve a woman's physical and mental health. It seems that some of the ingredients of semen can be absorbed into her body after sex and may improve breathing and control blood pressure. Two substances contained in semen – histamine and serotonin – are believed to have a beneficial effect on the womb and its muscles.

THE MECHANICS
OF AN ERECTION

In some animals the male penis develops an erection automatically whenever a female in heat approaches. But in humans it is not necessary for the female to be 'in heat'.

The reflex mechanism that enables a human penis to become erect functions more or less from birth. It is even common for babies who are no more than a day or so old to have erections as a result of an automatic erectile reflex – though it is not yet known what triggers this reflex or how it actually happens.

Just before puberty the ability of the penis to become erect increases dramatically, and it is perfectly possible for boys of nine or ten years of age to have serviceable erections.

In most adult men the development of an erection is not under voluntary control. (The exceptions are those yogi who have enough control over their bodies to produce erections by deliberate thought processes.) Sexual stimulation is the usual reason for the development of an erection and regular activity improves the efficiency of the reflex. A man who has sex often will find it easier to have an erection than a man who has sex only rarely.

Although the erection reflex is normally triggered only by sexual stimuli, it can be triggered by non-sexual stimuli in the right circumstances. A French sex expert has reported the case of a man who had sex a number of times in a room lit by a green light. Eventually the man automatically had an erection whenever he saw a green light. I rather suspect that this must have made driving in cities an exceptionally hazardous, if stimulating, adventure.

Normally, when a penis is limp the numerous arteries inside the organ are kept closed and empty of blood by tightened muscles in the penis. At the start of an erection the muscle fibres inside the penis become relaxed and loose, allowing blood to flow into the arteries and to fill the spongy tissues of the penis. The flow of blood into the penis compresses the veins which normally carry blood away from the penis, with the result that the penis gets rapidly larger. The penis rises into an upright position as it becomes firm because there is more of the spongy, erectile tissue on its lower side, and when this tissue fills with blood and expands it forces the whole penis upwards and into a shape and form better suited for sliding into the vagina.

It was at one time thought that a penis was either erect or non-erect but fairly recent research shows that the erectile state of a penis is constantly changing. The circumstances which help to create an erection are easily influenced by other factors, noticeably psychological ones such as fear, hope and embarrassment. On some occasions the penis will become erect against the will of, and to the embarrassment of, its owner. Yet on other occasions the penis will ignore attempts to encourage a response and will steadfastly refuse to become erect whatever entreaties may be made (and whoever makes them).

Once an erection develops it will usually last no more than two or three minutes. This may not sound very long but it is a lifetime compared to some animals. An elephant has an erection for around thirty seconds, while a chimpanzee's partner can expect a delay of only about ten seconds between the onset of an erection and ejaculation. On the other hand the human male is a sexual incompetent when compared to the male ferret – rather surprisingly this little animal is likely to have an erection lasting up to eight hours.

Most men have their greatest number of erections in their late teens and early twenties. Erections and nocturnal emissions of semen during erotic dreams (wet dreams) are an inevitable part of growing up, and teenage boys have sexuality thrust upon them whether they are ready for it or not.

Men over the age of thirty have a much greater chance of having a good erection in the morning rather than at night. There are three simple reasons for this: firstly, a full bladder is common early in the morning and a full bladder helps a man to produce a stronger erection; secondly, erotic dreams are more common in the early morning than late at night and thirdly, a good night's rest helps to give the older male a chance to build up his strength.

THE SCROTUM AND THE TESTICLES

The scrotum, which contains the two testicles, hangs below and behind the flaccid penis. It is a wrinkled sac of skin, which is flexible and extremely sensitive to touch, sexual stimulation and temperature changes. The two testicles normally hang at different heights, with the left one lower than the right. There is no complex physiological reason for this: it is simply to stop them knocking into one another.

The purpose of the scrotum is to enable the testicles to hang outside the body since they are extremely vulnerable to heat. When the outside temperature rises too much, the skin of the scrotal sac becomes looser – enabling the testes to move further away from the body and therefore remain cooler. When the outside temperature drops the scrotum contracts, pulling the testes

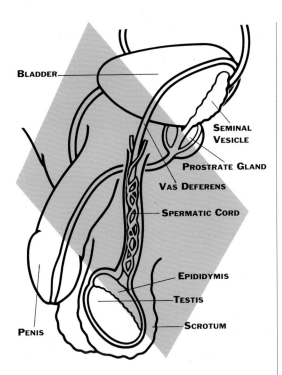

The testes hang outside the male body in a pouch of skin, known as the scrotum

closer to the body so that they can get warm. You can see this scrotal activity when a man gets into a warm or a cold shower.

In a male baby the testicles develop inside the body and usually move down into the scrotum before birth, but occasionally one or both testicles will fail to descend properly. This problem, which affects roughly one in every twenty boys, is called cryptorchidism, and either hormone treatment or surgery may be needed to ensure that the testicles do eventually descend into their rightful positions. If the testicles stay inside the body for too long, the high temperature can destroy the sperm producing tissues and this will eventually produce infertility.

Fear and sexual excitement can have the same effect on the testicles as cold weather. In children the testicles may go right up inside the body during moments of terror. Some Japanese fighters can still do this, and the trick is useful for professional wrestlers.

The two smallish, egg-shaped testicles inside the scrotum have two clear tasks: to produce

sperm and to produce male sex hormones. Each testis is attached to an epididymis where sperm are stored as they mature, and two tubes, the vas deferens, carry the sperm from the testes to the penis. En route, on each side of these tubes, there are storage sacs called seminal vesicles where mature sperm can be stored. Alongside the vas deferens are the glands that produce a fluid, which nourishes the sperm during and after a man's ejaculation.

ACTION MAN – THE ORGASM

As soon as a man becomes interested in sex he will usually have an erection. But an erect penis isn't the only sign of sexual arousal: his pulse and blood pressure will rise, his breathing rate will increase, he may acquire a skin flush, his testes will increase in size by as much as fifty per cent and will be pulled higher into his scrotum, his nipples will become erect, the muscles of his face will probably show some signs of tension and his buttock muscles will become tight and tense.

A few moments before ejaculation a few drops of a clear, sticky fluid will leak out of the end of the penis to moisten the glans and to prepare the way for the flow of semen which should follow. It is important to realise that these few drops of fluid may contain some sperm and can, on occasion, lead to a pregnancy.

At about the same time the seminal fluid which contains the sperm collects in the seminal vesicles which contract rhythmically, expelling their contents into the urethra at exactly the same moment as the prostate gland contracts and expels its secretions. A bulb in the urethra near the base of the penis more than doubles in size in order to provide the space to store these fluids for a few moments.

Once a male orgasm starts there is no way it can be stopped.

Strong contractions of the urethra and the prostate gland occur at intervals of just under a second, and the semen is forced out through the urethra with a considerable amount of force. The ancient Hebrews used to believe that if sperm didn't come out forcefully then it wasn't fertile and there is some sense in that. Sperm that leaves the penis forcefully will be more likely to reach the cervix and therefore, the uterus, where it will meet an egg. In older men semen leaves the penis with less force and, if unimpeded, is likely to travel a less spectacular distance. Most of the semen is usually forced out in just five or six spurts. Gradually, the contractions weaken and become less regular. Sometimes a few drops of urine may escape during all this physiological excitement – despite the existence of a valve designed to prevent such an occurrence. This small amount of urine will not do any harm.

Within a few seconds all the available semen will have been forced out of the penis and the ejaculation will be over.

At the moment of ejaculation a man's pulse rate, blood pressure and breathing rate will all reach a peak; any skin flush will deepen; his hands will clench; his facial muscles may go into spasm; his toes will spread and his whole body may become arched. Outwardly, the signs of orgasm in a man are similar to those in a woman.

Soon after the last drop of semen leaves the urethra, the penis – its job as sperm distributor done – will begin to wilt and lose its size. This process, known as detumescence, usually takes between a few seconds and a few minutes. In some animals small hooks hold the penis in place at this stage so that sexual intercourse will not end abruptly. There is no such aid on the human male organ and sexual interest often subsides rapidly – an occurrence that often gives rise to the complaint that 'he just rolls over and falls asleep as soon as he's finished'.

After ejaculation, the penis loses the blood that has filled it and provided it with strength and size. This happens because the arteries, which opened up as an erection developed, become constricted again with the result that no more blood can flow into the penis. The blood already in the penis flows out slowly at first, and then, as the tissues become less and less compressed, more

speedily. The collapse of an erection normally only occurs after ejaculation has taken place but it can occur if anything unpleasant or frightening occurs. A harsh comment, a sudden and distracting noise, a pain or a request to paint the ceiling can all lead to an almost instant disappearance of an otherwise satisfactory erection.

As the blood flows out of the penis, the testes begin to shrink and the scrotal sac lowers them down again. Blood flows out of the nipples, which get smaller, and any skin flush slowly disappears. The pulse rate drops, the blood pressure falls and breathing returns to normal.

A man cannot have another erection – or even get very excited sexually – after an orgasm has concluded and his penis and testicles may be extremely sensitive and tender to the touch. This is known as the 'refractory period' and is a stage of the orgasm that women do not have. The length of the 'refractory period' varies according to the individual's age and state of mind. Excitement, guilt or the ordinary stresses of everyday life can all have an influence.

In addition to the physical aftermath, it is also common for men to feel sad or even depressed after an orgasm, though the likelihood of this happening depends to a large extent upon the nature of the relationship. If the relationship is a satisfying and loving one then the man may be left with a warm, contented, happy feeling. But if the relationship is a one night stand then he may become depressed as he worries about risks and consequences.

It is quite common for men to feel so mentally drained and so physically exhausted after an orgasm that they have difficulty in staying awake. When young and making love to a new partner for the first time, a man may find it fairly easy to remain alert and interested, but when a relationship is a longer established one, a man may simply fall asleep.

If an erection does not lead to an orgasm, it is common for a man to be left feeling mentally frustrated. In addition he may feel some pain from prostatic engorgement.

HER

The visible sexual parts of a woman are known collectively as the vulva.

At the upper end of the vulva is an area known as the mons veneris or mount of Venus, which is named after the Roman goddess of love. The mons is made of a pad of fat which covers the hard pubic bone and acts as a cushion during intercourse, and is covered with a luxurious growth of tightly curled pubic hair which also has a cushioning effect.

Below the mount of Venus, the two outermost parts of the vulva are the labia majora, the outer lips of the vagina. These are made of elongated rolls of fat and are regarded as the female equivalent of the male scrotum. Like the mount of Venus they are also normally covered with pubic hair. It is a fact of life, but of virtually no practical significance, that the left labia majora is usually slightly larger than the right one.

Inside these two large, outer lips are the rather smaller, inner labia minora, delicate folds of skin which are usually free of pubic hair and which run parallel to the outer lips. These inner lips are normally closed together to seal the vagina off from the world. As with the labia majora the inner lips are often of different sizes. The colour of the inner lips often changes from a pale pink to a darker, rather rich, royal purple when their owner is sexually aroused. In some parts of the world a large pair of labia minora are considered to be the essence of true beauty.

The gap between the two inner lips is known as the vestibule, rather appropriately named since it is the entrance to the vagina. Just above the vestibule and underneath the mount of Venus the two inner lips meet to form a small, protective hood for the sensitive clitoris, the female equivalent of the male penis.

THE CLITORIS

The clitoris, like the penis, contains erectile tissue, which fills with blood and swells during sexual excitement. It also has a small covering rather like

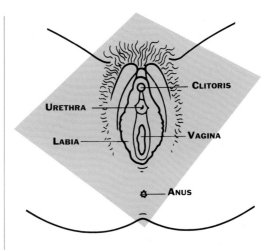

The collective name for the visible sexual parts of a woman is the vulva

a foreskin. The size and shape of the clitoris varies a great deal from one woman to another, but when unstimulated, the clitoris is usually no bigger than a pea. It contains numerous nerve endings and is exquisitely tender to the touch. Inch for inch, the clitoris is one of the most powerful, most responsive and most influential organs in the female body. Its sole function seems to be to provide sexual pleasure.

In some women the clitoris is stimulated quite naturally during ordinary intercourse: as the labia minora are pulled and pushed by the penis moving in and out of the vagina so the clitoris is gently massaged by the movement. Sometimes, however, the movement of the labial hood over the clitoris is not enough to produce an adequate sexual response and the clitoris may need to be stimulated directly – usually by the fingertips – although the clitoris is so sensitive that this has to be done carefully. When stimulated properly the clitoris gets bigger and much harder.

THE URETHRA

Just below the clitoris, at the top of the vestibule, is the opening of the urethra, the tube which allows the bladder to get rid of urine. Strong sphincter muscles, which can close together very tightly, ensure that urine only flows out of the bladder and down the urethra when it is

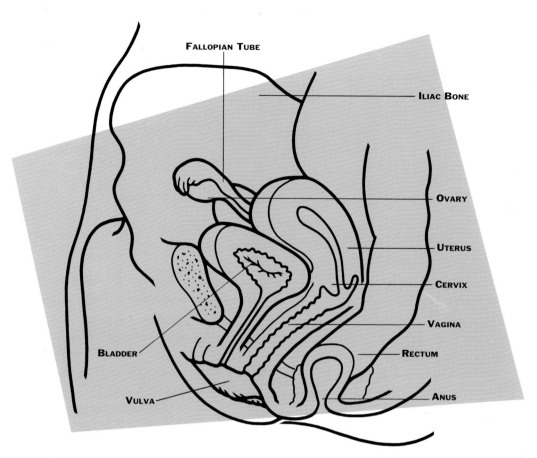

FALLOPIAN TUBE

ILIAC BONE

OVARY

UTERUS

CERVIX

VAGINA

RECTUM

ANUS

BLADDER

VULVA

appropriate but sometimes these muscles may relax a little during sexual arousal with the result that a few drops of urine may leak out. This may be embarrassing but is not harmful. Women who notice this problem can usually avoid it by emptying their bladders before having sex.

THE VAGINA

The vagina has three functions: to let the penis in (so that sperm can be deposited as close to the womb as possible), to allow a baby out, and to provide an escape route for the monthly menstrual flow. The vagina lies directly underneath the urethra and is a rather larger opening (though it is not unknown for the sexually inexperienced to mistake the urethral opening for the vagina, with disastrous consequences which include infertility and incontinence). The vaginal opening leads into a muscular tube three to four inches (7 to 10 cms) in length which stretches backwards and upwards towards the uterus or womb. In young girls who

are still virgins the opening of the vagina is often partly (and sometimes completely) sealed by the hymen, a thin sheet of skin which usually dissolves and disappears as a girl grows, leaving remnants around the vaginal entrance.

In some societies the existence of a hymen is, even today, regarded as evidence that a girl is still a virgin, and a bridegroom expects his new bride to suffer some pain and bleeding during intercourse as he stretches and then splits her hymen. The bridal sheet, dotted with a few spots of blood, is then triumphantly held up to the guests at the wedding reception, so that they can see both that the bride was a virgin and that the marriage has been consummated.

These days, however, most brides, whether or not they are sexual virgins, have little or no hymen left by their wedding night. The membrane may be split during bicycle or horse riding, during gymnastics or aerobics, or by the use of tampons during menstruation. It is not unknown for cosmetic surgeons to be asked to repair and re-install a tattered hymen, although these days in most societies it is perfectly acceptable for a bride to be hymenless. On rare occasions the hymen may be extremely thick and may need to be surgically pierced if consummation of a marriage or relationship is impossible.

Just inside the vagina there are two small pea-sized glands (one on each side) known as Bartholin's glands, which have the job of secreting fluid during sexual excitement in order to moisten the vaginal entrance and vulva. This fluid is needed to make it easier for the penis to enter the vagina.

In addition to the secretions from these glands, the walls of the vagina also produce lactic acid which helps to kill off any bugs which might get in from the outside world. Because the inside of the vagina is warm and moist and dark, it is an excellent breeding ground for infections of all kinds (see Chapter 9 for information on common vaginal infections). The production of lactic acid increases during a woman's reproductive years so that any risk of infection is kept to a minimum during the time that pregnancy might follow intercourse. Before puberty and after the menopause, the production of lactic acid secretions falls and, in addition to an increased risk of infection, there is also more likely to be soreness, dryness and pain during sexual intercourse.

The amount of moisture inside the vagina is increased by sexual excitement but happiness, fear and nervousness can also increase the quantity of secretions being produced in the vagina. There is also a slight increase in the amount of vaginal secretion before a menstrual period and a reduction during menstruation and this means that sex during a period may be dry and rather painful for some women.

The first third of the vagina is made up of a strong ring of muscles which enable the vagina to remain closed when not in use, and which give its owner the ability to grasp anything that happens to be inside it quite tightly. Women whose muscles have become slack because of childbirth can do exercises to strengthen them.

The overall size of the vagina is a subject of some concern both to men and to women. In some tribes in Africa, a man who is looking for a new wife will examine her first to check out the size and depth of her vagina. He may also want to see how well padded her mount of Venus is, and to check on the size of her labia.

Some women worry that their vaginas will be too small to accommodate an erect penis. This fear is usually groundless since the vagina can stretch enough to accommodate a baby's head. Other women, who may have given birth to several children, worry that their vaginas may have become too spacious. This fear is also groundless since the muscles within the vaginal walls can be strengthened to enable a woman to hold onto a penis of quite modest proportions.

The only real risk to do with size is that if a woman has a very small vagina and her partner has a very large penis, he may penetrate so far that the tip of his penis knocks into an ovary during sex. Since ovaries, like testicles, are well endowed with nerve endings this can be a very painful experience.

THE G SPOT

Although the clitoris is universally acknowledged as the source of sexual satisfaction in women, some researchers claim that there is also a small bean-shaped patch of erectile tissue attached to the inside of the top part of the vagina and situated an inch or two (2.5 to 5 cms) inside it. This area – known as the G spot – is said to be directly behind the pubic bone and one to one and a half inches (2.5 to 4 cms) across. It is known as the G spot after its discoverer Ernst Grafenberg, a German gynaecologist.

Grafenberg found the G spot during the 1940s when he was researching different methods of birth control. His claim that when stimulated by pressure the G spot triggers a vaginal orgasm substantiated previous, controversial claims that women can have two quite different types of orgasm – one triggered by stimulation of the clitoris, the other by movement inside the vagina.

In addition to producing an orgasm, stimulation of the G spot is also alleged to produce a fluid. It has been argued that the spot (or patch of tissue or gland) secretes a special fluid during orgasm and that women do, therefore, ejaculate when they reach a climax.

Despite all these claims there is still a considerable amount of scientific controversy among gynaecologists about whether or not the G spot really does exist, and whether or not it has any sexually active function. Pathologists report that they are unable to find the patch when dissecting dead bodies, but those who believe in its existence argue that this is because the G spot atrophies with age. Some experts, finding the existence of the G spot difficult to substantiate in the absence of any hard evidence, claim that the spot only exists in some women and that only a few women ejaculate.

There are a large number of gynaecologists and sex experts who do not believe in the existence of a G spot at all.

THE CERVIX AND UTERUS (OR WOMB)

The cervix or neck of the womb can be felt at the top end of the vagina.

The womb itself is hollow and shaped rather like an upside down pear – with the cervix where the pear stalk would be. The uterus consists of extremely strong muscles, which can stretch to many times their normal size for months at a time during pregnancy and then revert back to their original size afterwards. Every month the womb lining develops in order to provide a nourishing site for any egg which may be fertilized, giving it a chance to develop into a foetus. Since the womb is tucked well away inside a woman's body any developing baby will be protected by thick muscle and hard bone. The lining of the uterus, the endometrium, is under the control of hormones and the bleeding which marks the end of each menstrual cycle is a result of the endometrium breaking down and being discharged from the uterus.

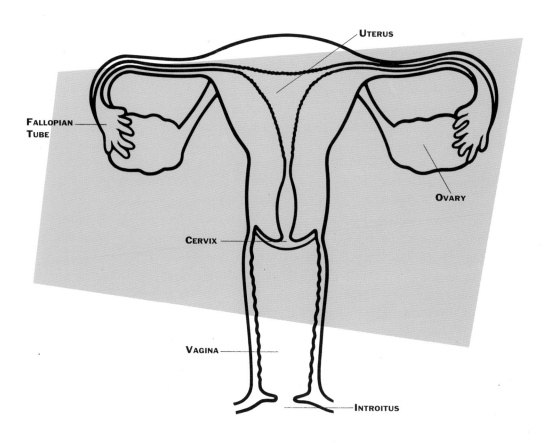

THE MIRACLE OF CONCEPTION

A woman can only have a baby when a male sperm meets a female egg.

Eggs, which are produced by the ovaries, reach the uterus by travelling along one of the two Fallopian tubes. The ovaries are the female equivalent of the male testicles; they manufacture the female sex hormones oestrogen and progesterone and store a supply of approximately half a million immature eggs.

Roughly once every twenty-eight days an egg will mature and leave the ovary ready for conception. Less than one in a thousand eggs will ever reach the uterus.

If sperm manage to get up the vagina, through the cervix and into the uterus at roughly the same time as an egg is released and available, then the sperm may fertilize the egg. If this happens then a baby will start to grow.

If there are no sperm handy when the egg is waiting then the endometrium (the special lining that the uterus develops every month in case a foetus needs supporting) is not needed and can be discharged as a monthly bleed. And the whole cycle begins again.

(See page 88 for further information about conception.)

ACTION WOMAN – AROUSAL AND ORGASM

The first sign that a woman is beginning to respond sexually, and that her body is preparing for intercourse, is when her vagina becomes moist with lubricating fluid. Lubrication usually starts quite quickly – usually within ten to thirty seconds of stimulation. (It is important to note, however, that lubrication of the vagina can also result from other types of stimulus, including fear, anxiety and general excitement).

Most of the lubrication comes from the glands at the entrance to the vagina but some comes from the walls of the vagina itself. When a woman is aroused, blood enters the tissues around the vagina in just the same way that blood flows into the penis of the stimulated man. The fluid that seeps out of the walls of the vagina has come from congested blood vessels.

While this is happening the clitoris is growing, again as a result of blood flowing into the area. The erectile tissue within the clitoris swells in exactly the same way that the erectile tissue in the penis swells. There are, in addition, changes in the breasts in this early phase of sexual excitement. The muscle fibres around the nipples contract with the result that the nipples become erect and increase in size as blood flows into them. The areas around the nipples – the areolae – become slightly swollen and in some women (particularly women who have never had children) the whole breast is likely to swell.

When a penis enters the vagina the physical presence of the male organ pulls on the labia minora so that there is some friction between the part of the labia that covers the clitoris (the clitoral hood) and the clitoris itself. Since the clitoris is packed with sensitive nerve endings – and is already swollen with blood – the response is often fairly fast and quite dramatic. The outer lips – the labia majora – open a little wider and become swollen, moving away from the vaginal entrance in order to give the penis more room. The labia minora also swell a little and, at this time, the vaginal muscles in the outer part of the vagina begin to expand.

In addition to these very specific changes in and around the vagina there are also some more general changes in a woman's body once sexual intercourse starts. The woman's pulse will increase, her blood pressure will rise and a red flush, rather like a measles rash, will appear on her breasts, chest and upper abdomen. Although, this sort of skin rash sometimes occurs in men, it is much more common in women, three-quarters of whom show some sort of rash during sexual excitement and arousal.

Sexual excitement in women (and in men) consists of three main phases.

The first phase is one of excitement and arousal (described above).

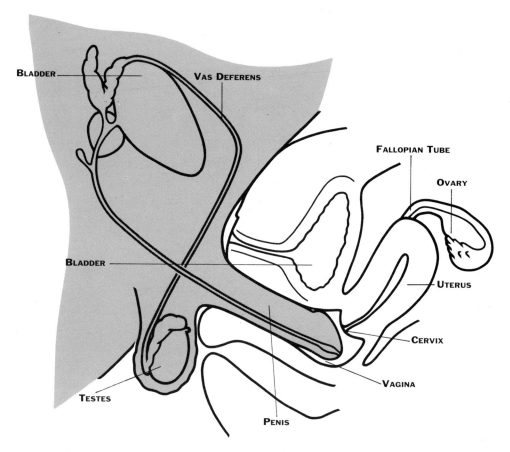

BLADDER — VAS DEFERENS

FALLOPIAN TUBE

OVARY

BLADDER

UTERUS

CERVIX

VAGINA

TESTES

PENIS

Cross-section of the penis penetrating the vagina during intercourse

The second phase is known as the plateau, during which the woman's body is prepared for orgasm. Her breathing rate increases, her pulse and blood pressure go up even further, any flushing that has already appeared becomes more noticeable and more widespread, and her face, hands and buttocks show signs of muscle tension. In the plateau phase of sexual excitement a woman's breasts, nipples and areolae will swell even more than before. Inside the vagina drops of fluid will ooze out from the Bartholin's glands and the tissues in and around the outer part of the vagina will swell. As the vagina tissues swell, so the vagina will grip the penis more and more tightly. The labia minora will darken in colour – going from pink to purple – and the clitoris will gradually become larger and more elevated.

The woman is now ready for an orgasm, the third and final phase of the excitement process.

There are many myths about just how women have orgasms and where they come from,

but an orgasm is an orgasm is an orgasm, and at the moment of truth it doesn't usually matter terribly *where* it came from or *how* it came about. There is, however, much discussion among sex experts about whether an orgasm can be triggered by stimulating the clitoris alone or whether stimulation of the vagina can also trigger an orgasm.

In cold, unemotional, clinical terms an orgasm is defined as a 'peak of sexual arousal which consists of uncontrollable muscle movements, a tingling, a general feeling of warmth and an indescribable sense of joy and pleasure'. One physiologist described an orgasm as a 'mass neuronal discharge, originating in a part of the brain between the amygdala and the hypothalamus'. During an orgasm most people, of both sexes, respond in much the same way and technically an orgasm is the same in women as it is in men. The following seven physical signs may be noticed during orgasm (but often only by a disinterested observer):

1. A PROGRESSIVE LOSS OF INTELLECTUAL CAPABILITIES.

2. DILATION OF THE PUPILS.

3. AN AGONIZED FACIAL EXPRESSION.

4. SHOUTING OUT LOUD – KNOWN AS INVOLUNTARY VOCALIZATION.

5. AN INCREASE IN THE PULSE RATE (RISING TO SOMEWHERE BETWEEN 120 AND 150).

6. AN INVOLUNTARY HEAVY THRUSTING MOVEMENT OF THE PELVIS.

7. CONTRACTIONS AND TIGHTENING OF VARIOUS MUSCLES AROUND THE BODY, RESULTING IN GASPING, TIGHTENING OF THE FINGERS, SPREADING OF THE TOES AND AN UPWARD MOVEMENT OF THE BIG TOE.

During a woman's orgasm the outer third of her vagina will usually contract rhythmically. A mild orgasm may be accompanied by three to five contractions whereas an intense orgasm will probably be accompanied by eight to twelve contractions.

When these pelvic contractions take place, some women say that they feel as if they are ejaculating. Others simply describe the contractions as a throbbing sensation which makes them feel warm all over. Despite the fact that the clitoris can be stimulated by the movement of the penis in and out of the vagina, most women do not have their orgasms directly as a result of sexual intercourse but need some additional manual stimulation. This inability to orgasm during sex often produces anxiety and guilt among women and men, who often feel that they have failed if they have to resort to such methods.

If a woman is fully aroused and sexually excited before penetration takes place, she may be able to reach an orgasm in as little as fifteen seconds. Normally, however, a woman takes rather longer: four minutes from start to finish is average. This is often considerably longer than a man can wait before he ejaculates and so his erection may start to lose its strength well before she reaches her orgasm.

When a woman has an orgasm the muscle tensions that have accumulated will slowly disappear. Blood will flow out of the labia, the clitoris, the nipples and the areolae and all those organs and tissues will shrink back to their normal size. The sexual flush will disappear from the skin (though many women do then begin to perspire, notably on their hands and on the soles of their feet), the vaginal muscles will return to normal and the clitoris will shrink and fall back downwards again to its previous position. At the same time as all this is happening, the opening in the cervix will expand slightly to give the sperm a better chance to swim through into the uterus.

The post-ejaculatory depression which affects men so much, does sometimes also affect women. It may help a woman who wants to get pregnant because by encouraging her to stay where she is – ideally flat on her back – it ensures that the semen will remain where it is, and not be displaced by any more movement or by muscle contractions resulting from more sexual arousal. Gynaecologists treating women who are trying to get pregnant usually advise them to rest – and to stay flat on their backs – after sex. Standing up merely makes life harder for the sperm.

Women who do not have an orgasm after being sexually aroused may, in addition to being left with a feeling of frustration and a lack of satisfaction, can be left with pain and congestion in the pelvic area. The blood vessels, which have swollen and filled with blood, do not empty quite so quickly when the first stages of orgasm do not lead to the final stage.

CHAPTER TWO

How To Turn Your Partner On

This chapter is designed for men who want to know what turns women on – and vice versa. Whether you are struggling to find a new partner or to revive a long established relationship that now has all the thrills and excitement of a pair of comfy old slippers, there are many things that you can do to make yourself more attractive sexually. And this does NOT mean making yourself look cheap or garish.

MAKE YOURSELF ATTRACTIVE

It is difficult for a woman to see her partner in sexual terms if she is used to seeing him crawling around underneath the car or mowing the lawn. And it is equally difficult for a man to see his partner in the way he saw her when they were courting if she is permanently hunched over an ironing-board or a sink full of dirty dishes.

So, here are some practical tips and hints! But do remember that these guidelines are very general. Although they are based on a large number of surveys and questionnaires, you should always try to wear clothes that make you feel comfortable and that suit you – and you should take into account your partner's preferences.

FOR WOMEN: HOW TO MAKE YOURSELF ATTRACTIVE TO MEN

CLOTHES

Clothes should be either loose, billowy and very feminine, or tight and figure-hugging, depending on your shape and what you feel comfortable in. Try to choose a wide variety of different clothes rather than variations on the same, ever popular theme. Try flowery, summer dresses, sleeveless and low cut. Or try a smart suit worn with a white blouse. Red and black are traditionally the most sexually provocative colours for clothes. Fabrics such as satin, silk and leather are sexier than cotton or wool.

Many men find a woman's curves sexy, and like to see women in figure-hugging clothes. Many others find loose clothing just as attractive – they can fantasize about the hidden figure.

HAIR

There are many clichés about what kind of hair men like. For instance, some women still claim that blondes have more fun. The best advice is probably to wear a style that suits you, and that you are comfortable with. Wax or shave your legs to remove the hair there and if you shave under your arms do so regularly – otherwise let it grow. Some men, although probably a minority, do like unshaven underarms.

SHOES

High heels may not be good for you but many men find them sexy, although if you look awkward, the effect will be comical rather than a turn-on. If you enjoy wearing high heels, do not be deterred if your partner is smaller than you.

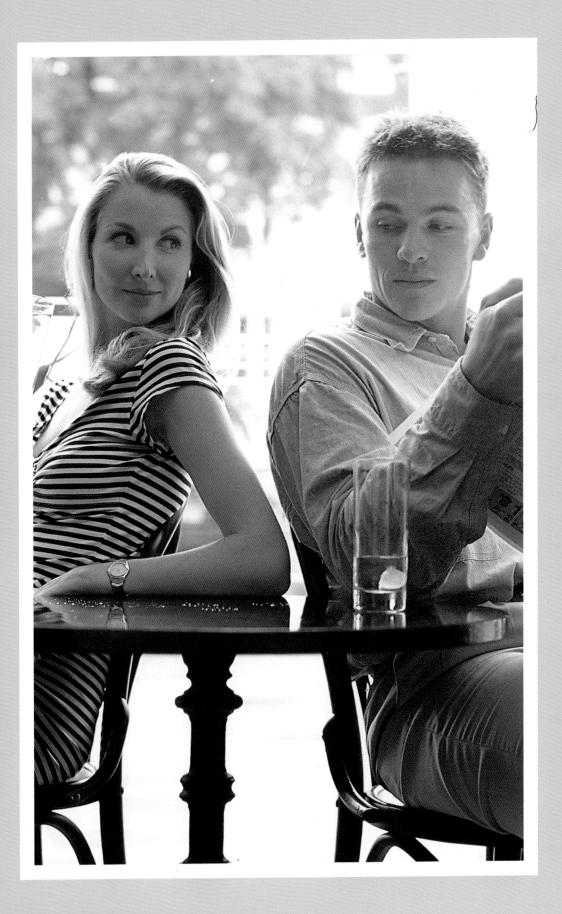

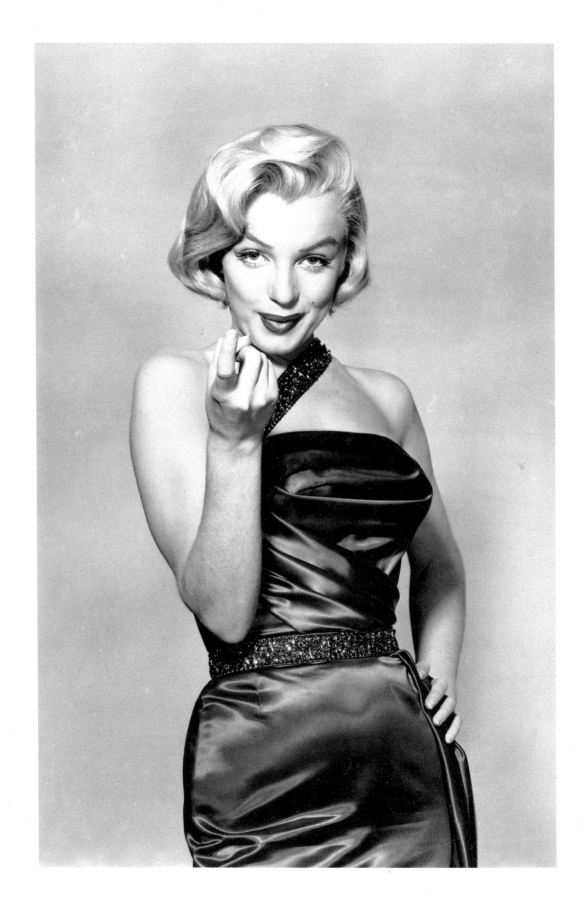

Accessories

Carry a small handbag, not a huge, capacious bag that makes you look over-competent. If you have attractive hands you can draw attention to them by wearing several rings on your fingers. If you want to draw more attention to your cleavage choose something bright to hang around your neck (a chunky necklace for example). If you wear a brooch it should be a bright one designed to draw attention to the breast upon which it is pinned.

Underwear

For a special evening, choose your underwear with him in mind. Try a lacy half-cup bra, skimpy lacy knickers and stockings and suspenders. They'll make you feel sexier and he'll love it. If you are feeling really racy, why not try stockings with seams? Black or white underwear is sensual, while red is unashamedly raunchy. And if you want to be certain of turning him on wear no underwear at all – and tell him just as you're going out!

Perfume

Many women use far too much perfume. A little perfume can be a turn-on, but too much can be a massive turn-off. Many men are allergic to perfume so too much can result in him wheezing and coughing all evening. Remember: we produce our own special, sexually attractive smells when we are sexually aroused. Those natural, human smells are really irresistible but if you use too much artificial perfume you'll drown them out completely.

The Way You Walk

Good posture, when walking or sitting, is very important – no one is attracted to a slouch! Also, unless you are very tall, try to make the most of your height and pull in your stomach and push back your shoulders as you walk in order to push out your chest. If you want to go a little further, you could try walking with a wiggle like Marilyn Monroe. However, make sure that you don't overdo it.

Your Eyes

If your man likes the made-up look then use make-up to attract attention to your eyes, which really are the window to your soul. Mascara and eyeliner will make your eyes look bigger and more irresistible. When you know he's looking at you look down for a second and then glance shyly up at him. Research shows that all things being equal most men automatically and instinctively choose the woman whose eyes have the biggest pupils. To make your pupils larger take a real interest in the people you meet – and in everything around you. Listen to what people say. Stay alert and awake. If you feel bored your eyes will give you away. Avoid bright lights too as your pupils will shrink when the lights are bright. If you wear spectacles try to take them

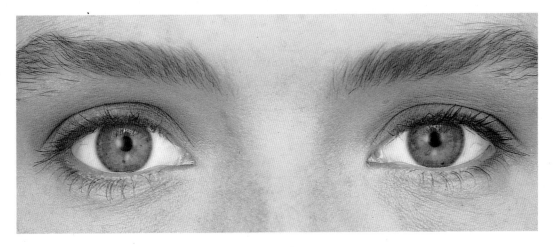

off when you meet the man you are trying to impress: spectacles seal off your eyes and make eye-to-eye contact difficult. But the very act of taking spectacles off can attract attention to your eyes, so don't worry about having to keep them off all the time. Just before you meet try fantasizing. It will make your heart beat faster, your face flush slightly and your pupils dilate. These subtle but real physical signs – produced by your own fantasy – will help to make you genuinely irresistible to the man you want to attract.

THE WAY YOU STAND AND SIT

Body language is vitally important: you can speak volumes by standing and sitting carefully. Stand with your body facing the man you fancy. You should stand with one foot pointing directly at him. If you want to accentuate the size, shape and prominence of your breasts push your shoulders back – otherwise lean forwards slightly so that you are as close to him as possible. Stand with one hand on your hip, or, if you have a belt, with a thumb tucked into it. When you sit, either have your knees pointing at the man you are interested in or else sit with your legs very slightly apart. Stroke your own legs and thighs occasionally and apparently carelessly to draw his attention to them. Hitching up your skirt an inch or two may sound corny but it works!

TOUCH AND MOVEMENT

Touch is a tremendous turn-on. It need only be the lightest of touches for the briefest moment. Let your fingers rest on his hand or arm for a second when you hand over a glass. Hold his arm lightly as you move through a crowd. Put your hand in his as you cross the road. And touch *yourself* constantly. Check your make-up, refresh your lipstick and tidy your hair regularly. When he sees you touching yourself, he will want to touch you too. Try a casual toss of your head to flick back your hair. If you are holding something (a cup or a plate) try holding it in such a way that you expose the inside of your wrist.

YOUR VOICE

If you're really feeling adventurous, you could try speaking in a slightly different voice when you want to project a sexy image. Lower your voice a little and try a rather husky tone. Do not attempt to speak in a little girl voice.

FOR MEN: HOW TO MAKE YOURSELF ATTRACTIVE TO WOMEN

CLOTHES

Slightly baggy, comfortable trousers are better than very tight ones, unless you are very young, perfectly formed and rather flashy. Choose clothes that make you look – and feel – relaxed. Light pastel colours and greens and browns are probably better than bright colours. Ties should be fairly plain but brightly coloured. If in doubt, the informal look is better than the formal look. Men should not look as though they've spent hours getting themselves ready.

HAIR

Whether you wear your hair long or short, wear it neat and clean. If tousled it should be a fairly controlled tousle. The first thing a woman examines when she sees a man for the first time is his bottom. The second thing she notices is his hair. Try to acquire a style that doesn't require too much effort – and never be seen using a comb. Avoid a beard, moustache, sideburns or designer stubble unless you're prepared to spend a lot of time on it. If you have a moustache, for example, it should be huge and shaggy and not small, neat and well-trimmed. Many women don't like the feel of kissing a man with a beard. And sideburns either look comical or indicate a man trying to recapture his youth.

SHOES

It is important that shoes are smart and clean. But apart from that, they aren't terribly important for a man. Solid shoes – especially brogues –

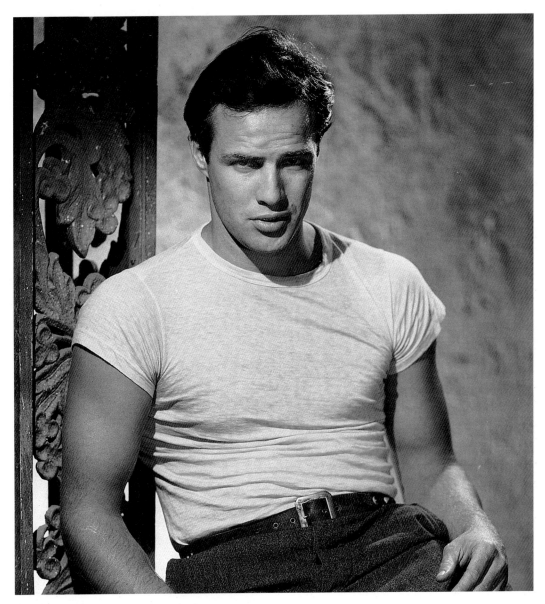

are better than trainers. If you need to wear higher heels to make you look taller make sure that they aren't obviously high or else you will merely attract attention to your lack of height.

ACCESSORIES

Avoid rings except for a signet ring or wedding ring. If you wear a belt choose something slim with a small neat buckle. Avoid broad belts with ornate, heavy fasteners. Avoid earrings. Your watch should have a traditional face; don't wear a digital watch. Don't have pens or a handkerchief in your top pocket. Never wear braces.

Avoid ostentatious cufflinks, button-down shirt collars and tie-pins, all of which make a man look too 'fussy'.

UNDERWEAR

Wear either skimpy briefs or boxer shorts – brightly coloured or patterned. Wear a T-shirt rather than a vest.

AFTERSHAVE

Don't drown yourself in aftershave or eau de cologne. While a little may be a turn-on, a lot can be a turn-off.

The Way You Walk

Pull in your stomach, stick out your chest and stand as upright as you can. Don't slouch – walk tall, with confidence.

The Way You Stand and Sit

Stand with your body facing the woman you are trying to make an impression on and with at least one foot pointing directly at her. Lean forwards slightly. When you sit down, keep your legs wide apart or your knees pointing directly at the woman you are interested in.

Your Eyes

Try to catch her eye and then hold her gaze for as long as you can. Look straight at her. Don't forget to smile.

Touch and Movement

Adjust and straighten your tie from time to time and try runing your fingers through your hair occasionally.

Your Voice

Lower your voice slightly and speak quietly, slowly and confidently.

Tip for Men and Women About What You Say

Be honest and passionate. Let your emotions show a little. Share your secrets (at least, the ones you are happy to share) and encourage your partner to confide in you. If you cover up your emotions you'll come across as flat and boring. Don't be afraid to speak out for things you believe in, but don't be controversial for the sake of it or start arguments, unless you're ready to see them through and prepared to see the end of a beautiful relationship! Genuine passion, sincerely voiced and spiced with a little humour can turn charm into charisma. If you aren't a good talker learn to be a good listener. Stay interested and show that you're interested by maintaining the all-important eye contact.

How Not to Turn Your Partner Off

Sometimes, when a relationship ends a man will say: 'I couldn't stand the way she was always late for our dates. That's what broke us up.' But it's not usually a particular habit that wrecks a relationship. It is far more likely to be a whole collection of character traits.

The Things That Turn Men and Women Off

1. Arrogance and an overbearing manner.
2. Thoughtlessness and rudeness.
3. Too much possessiveness and unwarranted jealousy.
4. Lack of a sense of humour.
5. Lack of patience and being over-critical.
6. Aggressiveness and violence.
7. Lack of personal hygiene.
8. Meanness.
9. Being boring and having no interests or enthusiasms.
10. Absence of emotional commitment.

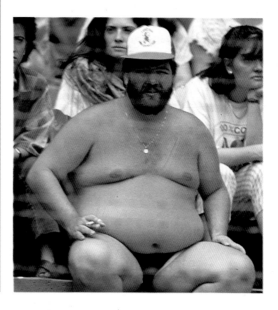

TWELVE THINGS ABOUT MEN THAT TURN WOMEN OFF

1. '...he never tells me he loves me...'

2. '...he never says I look nice...I don't want him to say I look beautiful, but the occasional compliment would be nice...'

3. '...he wears his socks and underclothes in bed and won't even take them off when we make love...'

4. 'he has an awful, overhanging beer belly and won't diet...'

5. '...he doesn't wash very often and when he does he doesn't do it very well...he smells...'

6. '...he has terrible bad breath...'

7. '...he comes in drunk and then wants to make love...'

8. '... he wears vast quantities of foul-smelling aftershave...'

9. '...he said he was in love with me but I'd only known him for an hour and I knew he was lying...'

10. '...he spends no time at all on foreplay...'

11.'...he can't have a kiss or a cuddle without wanting sex...'

12. '...he doesn't shave or cut his fingernails...'

TWELVE THINGS ABOUT WOMEN THAT ANNOY MEN

1. '...she spends hours getting herself ready and we're always late wherever we're going...'

2. '...she makes herself look gorgeous and then complains when I try to give her a kiss...'

3. '...she never wears the sexy lingerie I bought her for Christmas...'

4. '...she only ever wears make-up when we're going out...'

5. '...she wears hair rollers in bed...it's a real turn off...'

6. '...she never wants to try anything new or a bit different in bed...'

7. '...she's always making excuses for not having sex...'

8. '...she just lies there in bed while I do all the work...'

9. '...she never shows any interest in football or the things I like...'

10. '...she moans about the roof leaking just as I'm getting affectionate...'

11. '...she never tells me what she wants when we make love but always lets me know that she hasn't been satisfied...'

12. '...her breath always smells...'

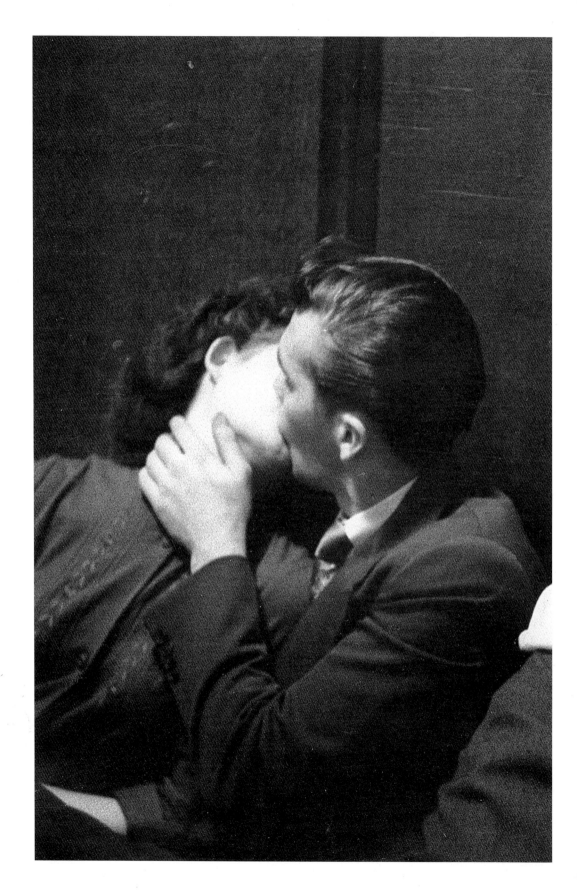

SEXUAL ETIQUETTE

THE RIGHT PLACE

Most of the time most people make love in their bedroom. But the bedroom isn't always the best place. Sometimes the walls may be too thin, so a couple may be inhibited by the thought that their every move, groan and gasp will be heard by the in-laws or the children. Noisy bedsprings and a door that doesn't lock can turn the most affectionate couple into celibates.

If your sex life has been crushed by family life, consider getting someone to look after the children for the weekend and then going away somewhere romantic where you can escape from blocked drains, piles of ironing, demanding children and thin walls.

Alternatively, why not have an evening of passion in the car? Many couples start their love life in the car but never even think about it again after they're married. And yet, despite the fact that gear levers and handbrakes are often positioned in such a way that they make excellent contraceptives, many couples find making love in the car liberating and enjoyable.

Or recapture the magic of your courtship by spending an evening out: an intimate meal in a restaurant and a cuddle in the back row of the cinema are excellent preludes to lovemaking.

If you are both bored with your sex life but have a home of your own then why not try making love *outside* the bedroom? There's the kitchen, living room, guest bedroom, hallway, garage or even the garden!

THE RIGHT TIME

The modern inventions of television and electricity have ruined sex for most people. Non-stop TV encourages us to stay up late and electricity enables us to keep warm without having a cuddle. It's hardly surprising that the biggest jump in the birthrate occurs nine months after every major power cut – when people rediscover the joys of things they'd forgotten.

Couples who try to make love late at night after a long evening in front of the TV set and an even longer day at work often discover problems. The man will probably have difficulty in getting a good erection and if he does then he'll either ejaculate quickly or not at all. Or he'll be so tired that he'll fall asleep whether his partner is satisfied or not.

The early morning is often a much better time. Sexual desire is often higher in the mornings and both partners may find it easier to get aroused. Best of all is a morning at the weekend when there's no rush to get to work. If you're worried about the children wandering in solve that problem by putting a lock or bolt on the bedroom door.

Or if early morning just doesn't seem right try going to bed earlier on in the evening. If you can't bear the thought of missing the TV and you don't have a video recorder, you could always plan your love-making around the programmes you want to watch.

SHOULD THE LIGHT BE ON OR OFF?

DIMB LIGHTS

Some people hate making love with the light on, while others find it difficult to get aroused with the light *off*.

Women or men who are shy about making love with the light on are usually either worried about their own bodies or worried about what

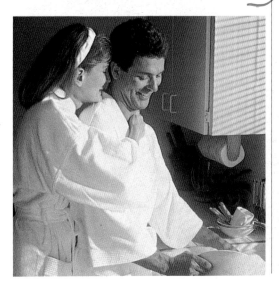

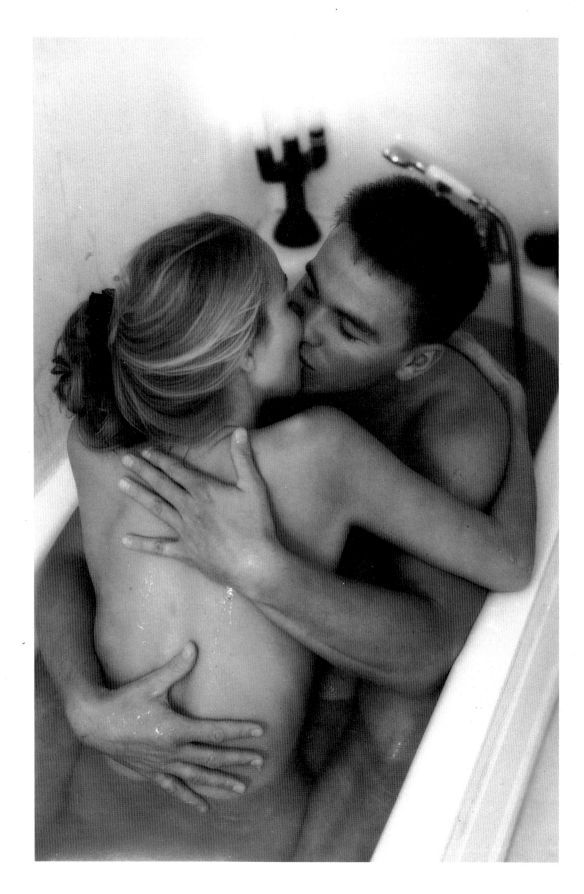

they'll see! Some married men and women have *never* seen their partner naked.

If you have opposing fancies try a compromise: put a low intensity bulb into a bedside lamp and fit it with a heavy shade or keep the lights on but make love under the duvet. The shy one among you may then be able to get accustomed to nudity bit by bit.

COURTSHIP AND FOREPLAY

One of the things most women regularly complain about is their partner's reluctance – or refusal – to spend much time on foreplay.

'I get really fed up,' is a typical female complaint, 'when my husband comes up behind me when I'm doing the washing-up and instantly wants to make love to me, whether I'm in the mood for it or not.'

'Nothing annoys me more,' is another, 'than getting into bed and suddenly finding him lying on top of me without a word of warning or the remotest attempt at seduction.'

It is usually men who are guilty of over-eagerness and a lack of understanding. But it isn't ONLY men. Some women are as guilty as the worst men, always wrongly assuming that men are permanently ready for action.

For both sexes foreplay is usually just as important as sex itself. There are exceptions, of course. Occasionally, a couple will want to plunge straight into steamy sex without any preliminaries. But this is usually either because the flirtation has been so successful that both partners are ready for sex or because the two partners have been separated for a long time. When this happens buttons will fly, material will rip and foreplay will seem entirely unnecessary.

However most people need to get into the mood to enjoy sex. And that means more than just a few moments of crude fondling. It means thought, care and tenderness. It often means forward planning or making the most of a quiet evening at home.

TEN TIPS FOR PUTTING SPARKLE BACK INTO YOUR LOVE LIFE

1. Make love out of doors.

2. Give each other a massage.

3. Dress up in your sexiest clothes, leave the house separately and then meet – as though by chance – in another part of town. Then pretend you are strangers who have just met for the first time.

4. If you normally make love with the light on try making love with the light off. And vice versa.

5. Take a bottle of champagne with you to bed.

6. Make love somewhere completely different: in the kitchen, on the patio, in the garage or on the landing.

7. Buy and then read together a raunchy book or magazine.

8. Take a bath or a shower together.

9. Look on pages 36 to 61 and then try some positions that you've never tried before. Or think up new positions that no one has ever tried before!

10. Beg, buy or borrow a polaroid camera and take photographs of one another.

THE IMPORTANCE OF TOUCHING

Touching is very therapeutic – and yet most of us do it far too infrequently. When small children are not touched regularly, they quickly become depressed and stop eating. A child who isn't touched can die of love starvation as truly as a child who isn't fed can die of food starvation. Children who are deprived of cuddles and love when they are small often grow up with deep-rooted psychological and emotional problems. They may become promiscuous in their constant, never-to-be-satisfied search for love.

Researchers all around the world have shown that it isn't just children who benefit from touching and cuddling. Insurance companies in America have found that if a wife kisses her husband goodbye when he goes off to work every morning, he will be less likely to have a car accident on the way to the office or the factory. He will, on average, live five years longer than if she doesn't give him a morning kiss. Without physical signs of affection we become more brittle, less emotionally stable and more susceptible to fear, pressure and distress.

Of course, touching isn't just reassuring. The right sort of touch, at the right time, in the right place, can be extremely arousing and stimulating. Some people imagine that the only place to touch one another during foreplay is immediately below the belt, but that is not true.

The average human body is covered with approximately two square metres of skin. Some of that skin contains areas of special sexual sensitivity – the genital areas and the lips are clearly erogenous – but *any* piece of skin on your body can become an erogenous zone if it is stimulated in the right way (see the box for tips on erogenous zones). The skin is an extremely complex organ of sexual response and communication.

Where do you start? It doesn't really matter. Both men and women tend to be very sensitive: To begin with try dragging your fingernails gently across your partner's skin. Move your fingers

- **ON AND AROUND THEIR NIPPLES**
- **IN AND AROUND THEIR NAVELS**
- **IN THEIR ARMPITS**
- **INSIDE THEIR UPPER THIGHS**
- **AT THE NAPE OF THEIR NECKS**
- **ALONG THE LENGTH OF THEIR SPINES**
- **ON THE INSIDE OF THEIR ELBOWS**
- **BEHIND THEIR KNEES**
- **ON THEIR BUTTOCKS**
- **AROUND THEIR EARS**

slowly and then quickly, in circles and in spirals. Stroke and massage every possible erogenous zone. Touch the stomach, the thighs, the backs of the knees and around the navel. Scratch the palms of both hands lightly with your nails. Blow in his or her ear. Kiss and then lick the most responsive spots and then blow on them while they are still wet. Penetrate his or her body symbolically by moving your finger rhythmically into and out of his or her navel, ear or mouth.

Learn to kiss properly. Relax your mouth, let your lips go limp. Then kiss everywhere that you have touched. Practise on the palm of your hand to see the difference between a hard, clenched kiss and a soft, thoroughly relaxed kiss. Brush his or her skin with your lips. Drag your lips along his or her most erogenous zones.

You may find that some areas are too sensitive for you to touch for long. A few women find that their nipples are too sensitive to be sucked.

Once you have worked your way around his or her body *then* you can move in on the predictably erogenous bits. For women, the clitoris is usually the most sensitive of all, followed by the inner lips of the vagina and then the outer lips.

For men the most sensitive part is usually the frenulum, the small piece of skin on the underside of the penis, where the glans meets the shaft, followed by the tip of the penis, the edge

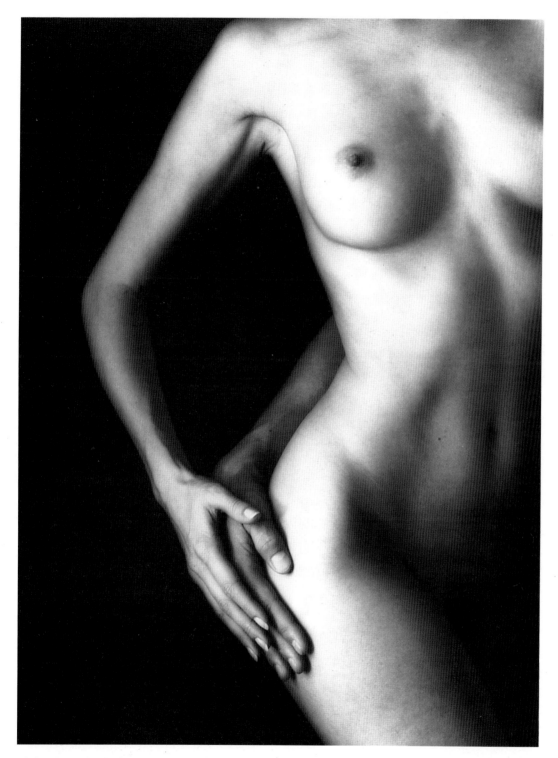

of the glans, the shaft and the testicles.

Both men and women are usually very sensitive in the area between their genitalia and their anus and both are also very likely to be sensitive to touch in and around the anus.

If you are shy about touching his or her sexual organs say so. Try touching very gently for just a second or two at a time. You will soon see the extraordinary amount of pleasure you can give with your fingertips.

CHAPTER THREE

Positional Play

There are scores – some would say hundreds – of different ways for a man and a woman to have sex together. Some of them are bizarre and uncomfortable and likely only to be used by those couples who are looking for the unusual and who are keen to work their way through the full range of sexual possibilities. Other positions may not appeal to all individuals but may be popular with some because they satisfy particular needs.

WHICH POSITION?

Different positions make it possible for people with different habits and preferences to obtain satisfaction. Some positions lend themselves to certain types of movement: pushing and thrusting, rocking from side to side, or grinding around in a circle. Others enable the woman to take full control or leave control in the hands of the male partner, if that is preferred.

On page 60 there is a chart designed to help you find the best position for your own – and your partner's – needs. But before that I have outlined the most popular sexual positions and their exciting variations.

THE MISSIONARY POSITION

The missionary position got its name many years ago when a group of white missionaries visited the South Sea Islands in the south-west Pacific. The islanders favoured a sexual position in which the man squats while his partner, lying on her back, wriggles her thighs over his and then pushes herself onto his erect penis. When they caught a glimpse of two of the missionaries making love, with the woman flat on her back and her husband lying on top of her, they found this highly amusing.

Despite the low opinion of the South Sea Islanders, the missionary position is an excellent way to make love and of all the different positions a man and a woman can get themselves into, it is probably the most widely known and used. As far as we know human beings are the only species to have sex looking at one another in the missionary position (most animals use the rear entry position).

The immediate advantage of the missionary position is that it is easy to get into. You don't have to be a contortionist. You don't even have to be super-fit or super-flexible. She lies down, usually with her legs apart, and he lies down on top of her with his legs inside hers. If a couple are of roughly similar height then they will be perfectly positioned. The man will be able to slide his erect penis into the woman's vagina and they will be able to see one another and kiss and hold one another.

Some women dislike the position if their partner is large or heavy, claiming that even if he takes some of his own weight on his elbows they still feel uncomfortable or suffocated. Some feminists object to the position, saying that it puts the woman into an inferior and submissive position which is a physical metaphor for society. But here are some reasons why so many women and men prefer the missionary position to the many others possible positions.

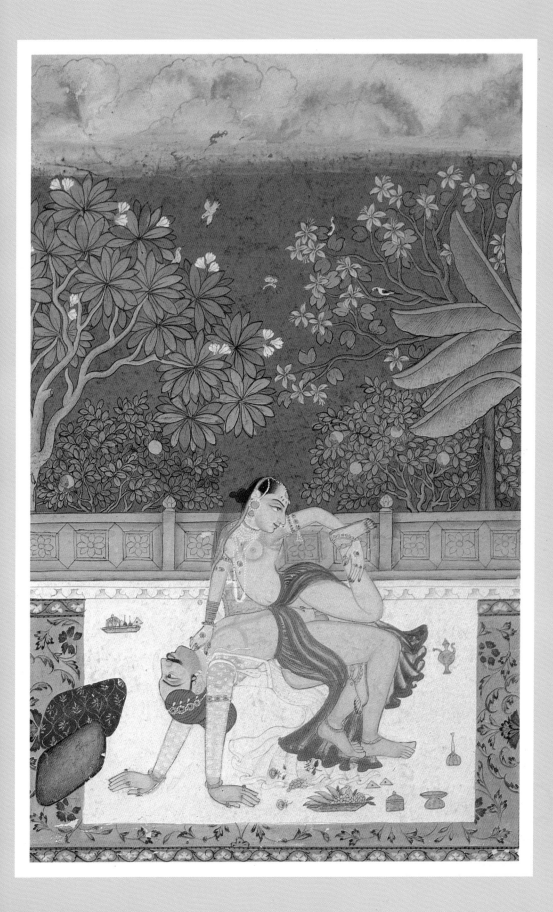

WOMEN LIKE THE MISSIONARY POSITION BECAUSE:

1. They find that it gives them a good orgasm. Many women who like to take a dominant role in sex enjoy the missionary position because it provides their clitoris with the sort of stimulation that enables them to have a satisfying orgasm. A woman in the missionary position can set the pace and can respond quite actively. By spreading her legs wide she can move her hips and her pelvis and if she keeps her feet flat on the bed and bends her knees she will be able to thrust herself against her partner. She can use her hands too; reaching behind him to caress or scratch his back and buttocks or reaching down between their bodies to hold his penis or to touch her own clitoris.

2. They like to be controlled during love-making. Some – but certainly not all – of the women who like the missionary position are passive. They prefer to be made love to by a strong man who will make all the moves and who will determine the pattern of movement and the tempo during sex. They like to lie fairly still.

The missionary position enables some women to enjoy what is happening to them without feeling that they have too much control over it. Women who tend to feel guilty about sex can enjoy the physical sensations without too many mental anxieties.

3. It enables them to look at their lover.
The missionary position is one of the few positions that enables both partners to look into one another's eyes and to kiss whenever they want to. Many women claim that they get most emotional pleasure out of the missionary position.

MEN LIKE THE MISSIONARY POSITION BECAUSE:

1. They can be in charge. Many men like to feel in charge and the missionary position makes them feel masculine, dominant and aggressive. Men who have doubts about their masculinity

do not like positions in which a woman takes a dominating role, and so for them the missionary position is perfect.

2. They can see, touch and caress their partner. The missionary position enables a man to look at his partner, to admire and fondle her breasts, and to kiss her and look into her eyes.

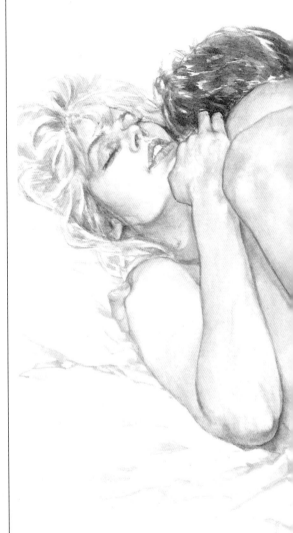

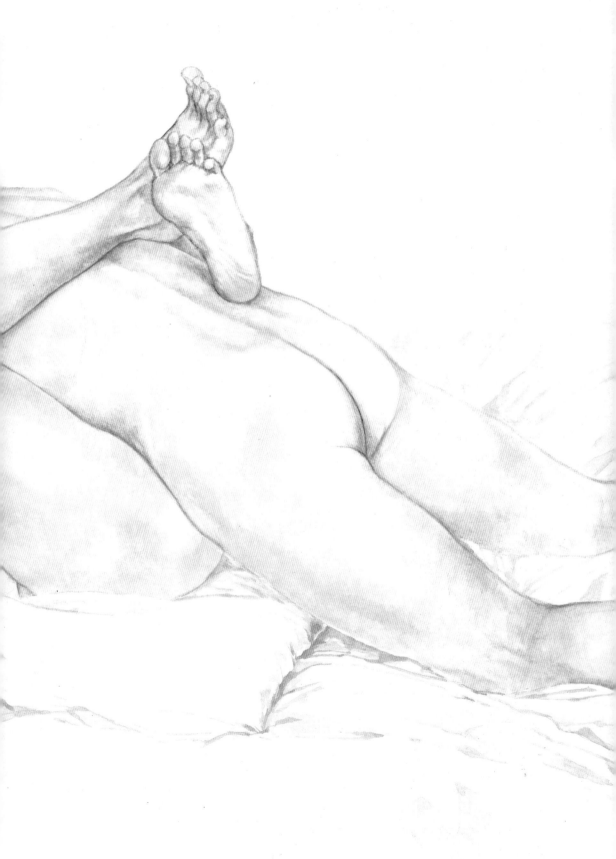

VARIATIONS ON THE MISSIONARY POSITION

Some of these variations offer specific advantages. Others are probably best kept for a wet Sunday morning when you've tried everything else and are prepared to end up lying on the floor laughing. I have listed only the most basic variations. If you have the time and the imagination you will undoubtedly be able to think of dozens of additional variations of your own!

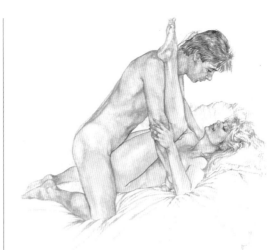

Variation 1

Instead of having both his legs between her thighs, the man has one leg outside her thighs and the other in between them. This position is called 'flanquette'. The main advantage of this position is that it produces extra contact between the penis and the clitoris, so women usually find it easier to reach orgasm. Another advantage is that both partners have greater freedom of movement. She can raise one hip slightly off the bed and move her pelvis more freely. He may be able to take most of his weight on one side, giving him a chance to use one hand to caress her body.

Variation 2

She lies flat on her back and lifts her legs straight up into the air so that her feet are pointing at the ceiling. He then kneels and moves as close to her as he can and she lowers her legs onto his shoulders. Both partners can see one another, but there is relatively little skin contact. He can't fondle her because he has to hold her to him and unless she has very long arms she won't be able to fondle him. He is in total control. The advantage of this position is that he can get his penis a long way inside her. Some men like this variation because it makes them feel powerful. Some women enjoy the deep penetration.

Variation 3

The woman gets into the ordinary missionary position but slips a pillow underneath her bottom before he lies down on top of her. The pillow changes the position of her pelvis and makes it easier for her to have an orgasm. The pillow also makes this position more comfortable for women who are slim or have small buttocks.

Variation 4

She begins by lying flat on her back with her legs wide apart. He kneels between her legs, puts both hands underneath her bottom and lifts her up off the bed. She wraps her legs around his waist. He

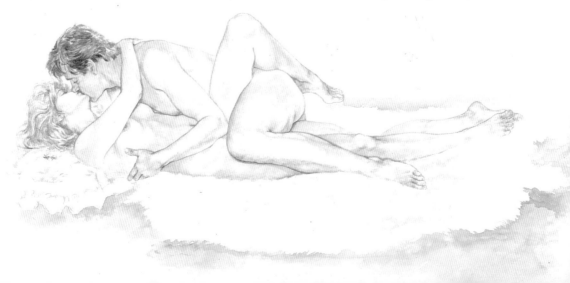

then enters her. Neither partner has much freedom in this position and there is little opportunity for kissing or fondling. He has control and a good view of what is going on.

Variation 5

She lies on her back with her legs open and slightly raised on the bed, and the man lies diagonally across her. He then enters her and rocks gently from side to side. The woman has some control: she can use her hands to guide the tempo of his rocking movements.

Variation 6

She lies on her back with her legs raised straight up in the air. He lies on his side at right angles to her, with his head sticking over one side of the bed and his feet hanging over the other edge. He then enters her. Neither partner can really see what is going on. But, technically, he is on top of her so this is a variation on the missionary position.

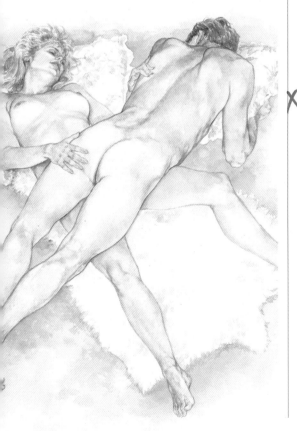

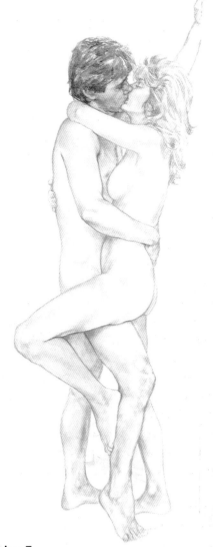

Variation 7

In most of these variations at least one partner is usually horizontal. But both partners can be vertical – as in this variation. She stands up and leans against a wall, tree or some other sturdy object. He then stands in front of her, pinning her to the wall and enters her. Unlike the basic missionary position, both partners are completely free to use their hands. This position is only really suitable if both partners are of a similar height. Otherwise, the shorter of the two may need a couple of telephone directories! There are several variations on *this* variation. The most obvious involves her wrapping both her legs around his waist and being held in his arms. Less dramatically she can wrap just one leg around his waist.

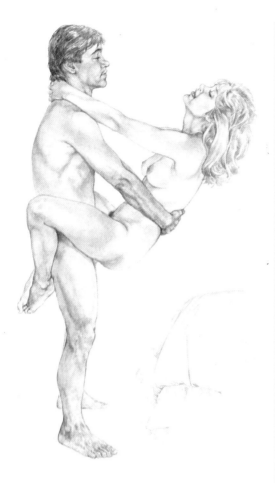

THE WOMAN ON TOP POSITION

In the basic 'woman on top' position, the male partner lies flat on his back and the female partner kneels above him and lowers herself down onto him. She has total control of the depth of penetration. This position, the most passive for a man and the most active, assertive and dominant for a woman used to be popular in Ancient Greece and has always been very popular in the Orient.

WOMEN LIKE THE WOMAN ON TOP POSITION BECAUSE:

1. She can take control. Being on top enables the woman to control the depth to which his penis enters her and the speed and rhythm of their love-making. She can move up and down, or round and round, or from side to side. She can lean forwards, kiss him, dangle her breasts in front of his face or hold both his wrists above his head so that he is in a submissive position. She can lean backwards and take herself out of reach. She can reach down to touch his penis and can take herself to orgasm manually; she can stimulate her clitoris and keep herself close to orgasm for long periods of time. Many women claim that they get more – and better – orgasms in this position. Women who like to remain in control, who are afraid of being dominated, who like to be able to move freely and to assert themselves prefer this position.

2. She can see what is happening. In this position she can see him enter her.

MEN LIKE THE WOMAN ON TOP POSITION BECAUSE:

1. It means less work for them. Men who have been ill (or who are still ill) prefer this position because it enables them to lie relatively still and hand over the responsibility for active movement to their partner.

2. Being a passive partner is different. Most men are accustomed to taking the lead in sex. They may find taking a passive role to be an exciting and stimulating experiment.

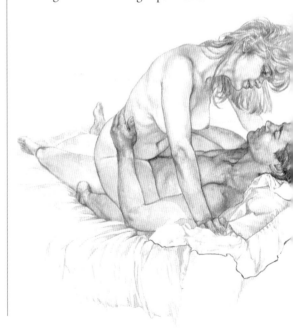

3. They can see exactly what is happening. The woman on top position is one of the few positions which enable a man to watch a woman as she approaches orgasm. This is a position in which he can touch, kiss, suck and play with her breasts and nipples while making love.

4. Intercourse is usually prolonged. A good erection is needed to enter a woman in this position but once inside intercourse is likely to be prolonged. Men who suffer from premature ejaculation may prefer this position.

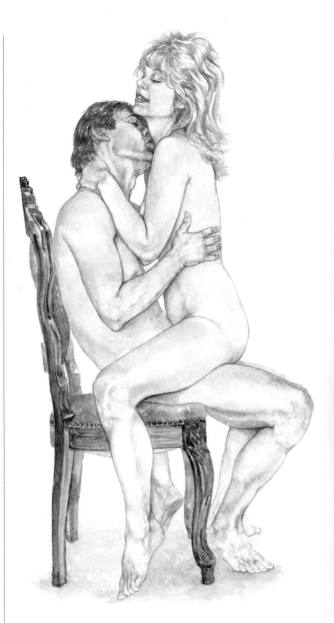

NOTE

SOME COUPLES PREFER TO START WITH THE 'WOMAN ON TOP POSITION' SO THAT SHE CAN HAVE HER ORGASM FIRST. THEN THEY REVERT TO THE MISSIONARY POSITION SO THAT HE CAN CLIMAX. THE ADVANTAGE OF THIS IS THAT IT ENSURES THAT HE DOESN'T FALL ASLEEP IMMEDIATELY HE HAS HAD HIS ORGASM. SHE GETS A CHANCE TO HOLD HIM FOR A WHILE AFTER SHE HAS HAD HER ORGASM.

VARIATIONS ON THE WOMAN ON TOP POSITION

There are a number of variations on the woman on top position. Remember that because this position originated in the East, some variations are best suited to individuals who are rather smaller and more agile than many westerners are. Large lovers may find some of these positions painful, impossible or simply unsatisfying.

Variation 1

The most obvious variation is for her to face away from him. This means that they cannot see one another or kiss. He cannot easily touch her breasts. She, however, has even more control than usual. She can still see what is happening,

can touch and fondle his scrotum and control the movement on her clitoris.

Variation 2

He sits on an ordinary dining chair. Facing him she then sits astride him. Both partners can touch, caress and kiss. This position requires little effort by either partner. She has most control and penetration is not deep.

Variation 3

He kneels and then leans back with one or both of his hands behind him. She faces him and then

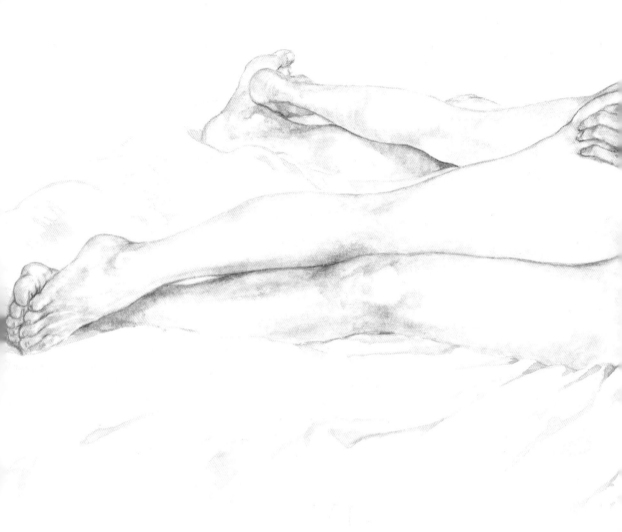

moves her bottom between his thighs, so that she can push herself onto his penis. She can drape her legs over his knees. She will have to stretch her arms out behind her to stop herself falling backwards. Neither partner will be able to use their hands and there is relatively little skin contact in this position but both partners can see exactly what is happening. Since the woman is still on top she still has control.

Variation 4

He lies on his back and she sits astride him as before. The only difference is that she has both legs on the same side and is, therefore, sitting 'side saddle'. She will probably need to balance herself by putting her arms behind her and taking some of her weight on her hands on the other side of his legs.

Variation 5

He kneels and sits up straight. She squats with her thighs parallel to the ground and balances on the balls of her feet. She then lowers herself onto him, holding onto him to keep herself steady. He can put his hands underneath her bottom to help. Even though she probably needs to hold on she can keep one hand free so that she can fondle him. She still has almost total control.

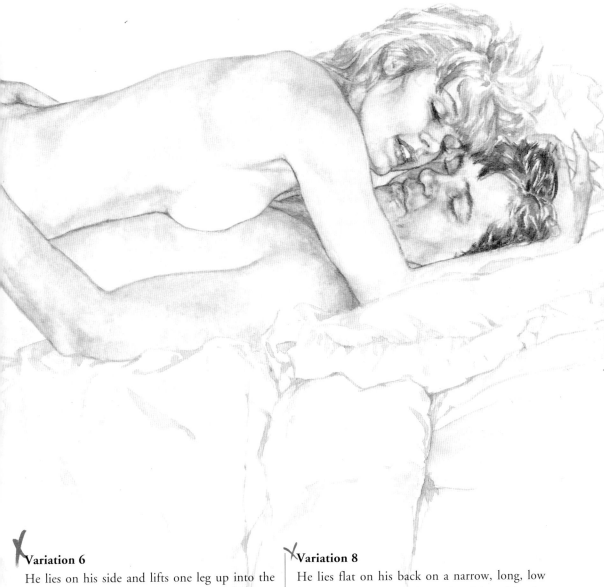

Variation 6

He lies on his side and lifts one leg up into the air. She then kneels astride his lower leg and lowers herself onto him. She is in total control.

Variation 7

He lies flat on his back with his legs open and she lies on top of him with her legs over his legs and her feet over his feet. She rests her arms on her elbows on either side of his shoulders. She has total control of the tempo of lovemaking by using her elbows to move herself up and down against her partner. She can vary her position by closing her legs tightly.

Variation 8

He lies flat on his back on a narrow, long, low table. With one leg either side of the table, she lowers herself onto him. Depending on the height of the table, she can either squat or remain half-standing

Variation 9

He sits with his legs apart. She faces him and then edges forward and puts her legs around his body. She then lower herself onto his erect penis. The advantage of this position is that both partners can hold and caress and kiss one another freely.

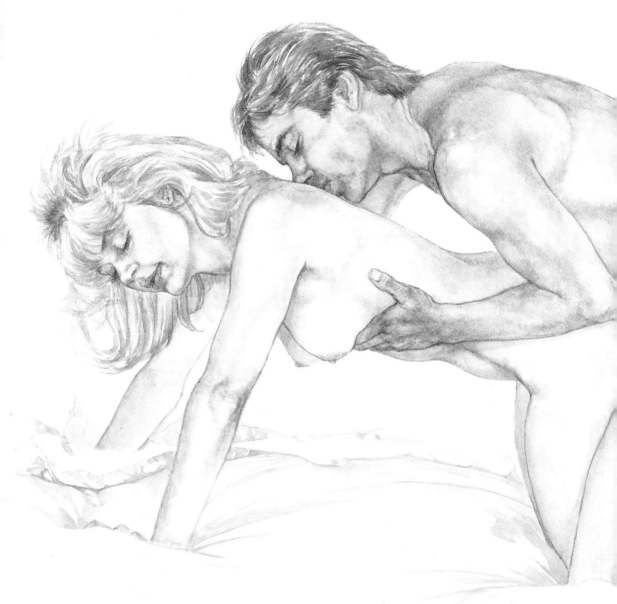

REAR ENTRY POSITION

The rear entry position (known to the French as 'croupade') is very popular. It is one of the most natural sexual positions and is the sexual position used by most mammals as the only option.

She kneels down and supports her shoulders by putting her hands on the floor. Her back should be horizontal to the floor. He approaches her from behind and uses a hand to guide his penis into her. He may be kneeling or squatting or may even sit astride her, like a jockey on a horse. She has no control over what is happening and unless she looks over her shoulder she can see nothing. He can see everything, and if he leans forwards he can touch her breasts and her clitoris. It is possible for him to penetrate her very deeply from this position and he can get maximum penetration by sitting astride her and gripping her thighs with his thighs. Deep penetration is so easy in this position that he must be careful not to push too hard or he may hit an ovary, which can be extremely painful.

If she finds this position tiring, she can build up a pile of cushions beneath her. Or she can kneel on the floor and rest her arms on a bed.

MEN LIKE THE REAR ENTRY POSITION BECAUSE:

They have control.

For men this is probably the most assertive of all positions. It is a position traditionally used by Eskimos, where the lack of face-to-face contact is an advantage in a society where men loan out their wives to honoured guests. Men who prefer to initiate and dominate sex prefer this position.

VARIATIONS ON THE REAR ENTRY POSITION:

Variation 1

She lies face downwards on the floor. He then approaches her from behind, putting one leg between hers. This is the reverse of the frontal 'flanquette' position and is known by the French as 'cuissade'.

Variation 2

She lies on her side and he puts both his legs in between hers. She then lifts her upper leg, swings it round and curls it around the back of his thighs. The movement means that he can see as well as fondle her breasts.

Variation 3

He lies on his side and she backs her bottom towards him. Her legs are at right angles to her body and her feet are by his face. There is very little visual or manual contact for either partner.

Variation 4

She lies flat on her back on the floor and lifts her legs so that they almost touch the floor beyond her head. Her vagina is very clearly exposed, which her partner will probably find very exciting. Facing away from her he then lowers himself into a sitting position and pushes his penis into her. This is a very detached position since neither partner can even see the other, although entry is relatively easy. Since this position produces very deep penetration it should be tried with caution.

WOMEN LIKE THE REAR ENTRY POSITION BECAUSE:

She has no control.

For women this is the most submissive and impersonal of positions. Unless she looks over her shoulder or has a mirror positioned in front of her, she cannot see her partner and she has no control over what happens. Women who like to maintain an emotional distance or like to let their partner take control during sex prefer this position to any other, as do women who enjoy deep penetration.

Variation 5

He kneels and then falls back to support himself with his arms behind him. She kneels and faces the same way as him. Keeping her legs apart she backs towards him. Her legs go outside his knees and her vagina eventually meets his penis. The man is unable to caress his partner.

Variation 6

She lies with her chest and head on a table. He approaches her from behind, lifts her legs up and enters her from behind, holding her legs on either side of his body.

Variation 7

She stands a yard away from a wall or piece of furniture and leans forward so that her arms and head are supported. She has her legs wide apart. He then approaches her from behind.

Variation 8

He leans with his back against a wall and his feet about a yard away from it. He may need to bend his knees if he is much taller than her. She then backs onto him. This is the only rear entry position in which the woman controls the movement and the penetration.

Variation 9

She kneels in the standard rear entry position but instead of kneeling behind her he bends down and picks up her legs. She supports her outstretched body on her arms. He then pushes himself forwards slightly so that his penis enters her. Penetration can be quite deep but there is little emotional contact and no opportunity for physical caresses.

Variation 10

Instead of kneeling, she lies on her side and he, also lying on his side, approaches her from behind. This position is gentle rather than aggressive and is very suitable for partners who are ill or convalescent, and for women who are pregnant. Men who can only get weak erections will find that this position enables them to enter their partner very easily, while men who are partially impotent may be able to regain their confidence by using it. This position is also suitable for the overweight.

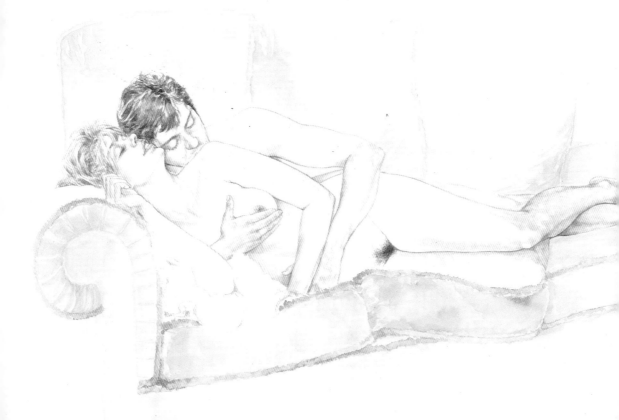

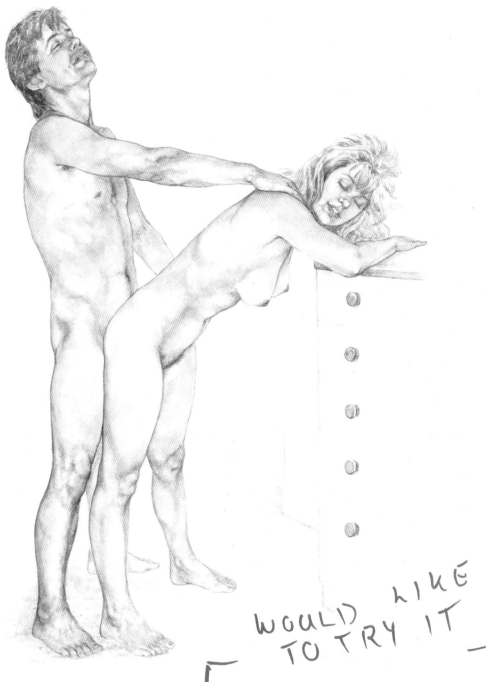

WOULD LIKE TO TRY IT

THE SIDE BY SIDE POSITION

Making love side by side is the most democratic of positions. Both partners face one another and because both pairs of legs have to be entwined to make penetration possible, there is inevitably strong skin contact. Neither partner is dominant, neither is submissive. Both partners can touch and caress and kiss one another. This position is peaceful, restful, physically undemanding and emotionally rewarding.

ORAL SEX

Oral sex is a natural, healthy practice which millions regard as an enjoyable variation on other forms of sex. Oral sex involving a mouth and the female sexual organs is known as cunnilingus. Oral sex involving a mouth and the male sexual organs is known as fellatio.

The mouth is well designed for sex. The shape of the mouth, the lips and the tongue mean that stroking, kissing, licking, probing and penetrating are all possible. The mouth is equipped with nerve endings and taste buds that enable the person performing oral sex to taste the juices which emerge from the vagina or penis.

Many sex books discuss position 69 in which both partners perform oral sex on one another simultaneously. (To see where the position got its 'number' just look at the number!) The advantage of this twin position is that both partners are fully involved. But there are two main drawbacks. The first is that a partner who is approaching an orgasm may find it difficult to concentrate on what he or she is doing. The second drawback is that the position can be quite uncomfortable and difficult to get into.

It is usually easier to take turns at enjoying oral sex and usually better if the woman is on the receiving end first. Apart from sheer gallantry, there are two simple reasons for this. First, women usually stay in the mood for sex after they have had an orgasm whereas men are prone to fall asleep. Second, he will probably find that his erection develops while he is performing oral sex on her.

Although oral sex is very popular – and widely performed – some people are frightened of it. Women fear that they may choke, they worry about having something as large as a penis in their mouths and they may be alarmed at the prospect of him ejaculating in her mouth.

If one partner is shy or hesitant then it is important that the other partner does not push things along too quickly. An introduction to oral sex can begin with a simple genital kiss, keeping the lips closed. Then, if both partners are willing and eager, progress can be made a little at a time on subsequent occasions.

It is usually thought that the person doing the sucking or kissing is adopting a passive or submissive role but in fact either partner can be dominant. When a woman is performing fellatio on a man she will be dominant if he is lying and she is above him. On the other hand if he is standing while she is kneeling and he holds her head while she performs fellatio then he will have much more control.

CUNNILINGUS

Women who want their partners to perform cunnilingus should make sure that they wash thoroughly beforehand. It is irresponsible to expect a partner to perform cunnilingus if there is any infection present.

The clitoris is the most sensitive part of a woman's body. And it is extremely tender. Be careful with teeth and nails. It is often better to begin by kissing the labia minora and the entrance to the vagina. You can then run your tongue along and around the vaginal entrance. Stroking, kissing and touching will be more enjoyable for her than prodding, pushing or squeezing. You may like to try sliding your tongue into her vagina. Most men find the acid taste of vaginal juices exciting. It is best to kiss around the clitoris rather than to kiss it directly.

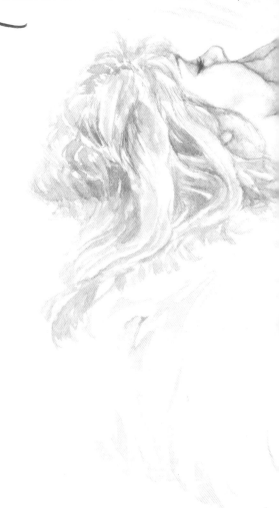

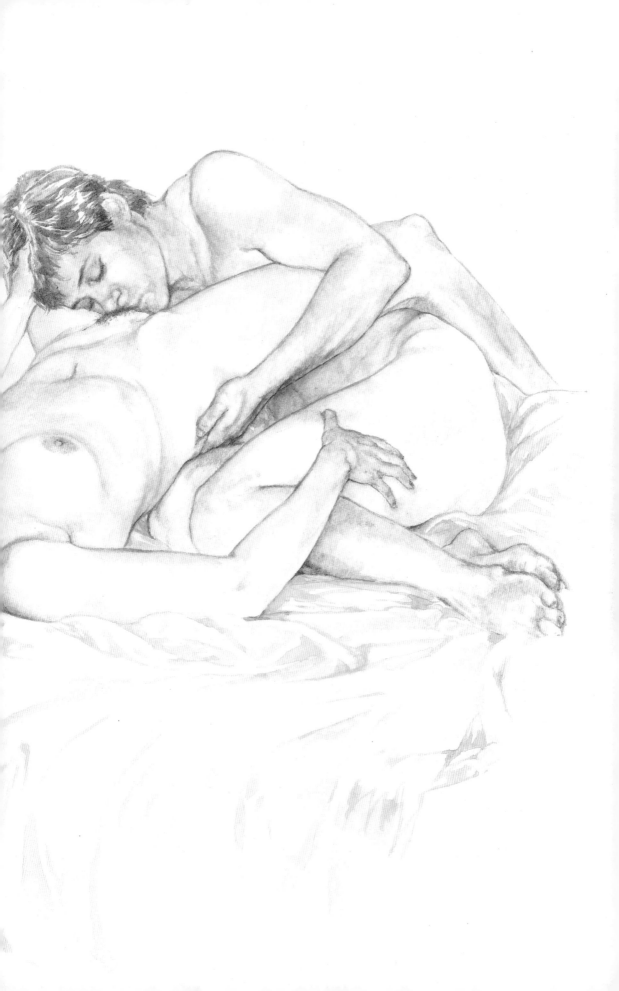

FOUR POSITIONS FOR CUNNILINGUS

1. He lies on his back on the floor or bed. She gently lowers herself down onto him until her vagina meets his mouth. If she faces his feet she can use her hands to touch and caress his penis. If she is very flexible she may be able to lower herself forward to perform fellatio on him at the same time.

2. She sits on an ordinary chair. He kneels or squats in front of her. She moves to the front of the chair so that her vagina is exposed and close to his face.

3. She lies on her back with her knees drawn up towards her chest. He approaches her lying on his side. If her legs tire she can lower them so that her feet touch the floor on the other side of his head.

4. He sits on a chair. She lies on her back on the floor in front of him. He bends down and picks her up so that her back is resting on his knees. She moves her legs so that they are over his shoulders. By now her vagina will be close to his mouth and her head will be hanging down. If she doesn't weigh too much and she can stand the fact that the blood will rush to her head this is a good position.

TWO WARNINGS

1. SEXUALLY TRANSMITTED DISEASES (IF PRESENT) CAN BE TRANSMITTED TO THE MOUTH AS EASILY AS TO THE PENIS.

2. IF CUNNILINGUS FOLLOWS FELLATIO AND KISSING IN THE RIGHT ORDER THE RESULT CAN BE CONCEPTION! (HE COMES IN HER MOUTH, SHE PASSES THE SEMEN TO HIM IN A KISS AND HE DEPOSITS THE SEMEN IN HER VAGINA FROM HIS MOUTH). THE CHANCES OF THIS HAPPENING ARE SMALL.

FELLATIO

Men who want their partners to perform oral sex on them should make sure that they wash thoroughly beforehand. Men who are uncircumcised should roll down their foreskins and clean underneath. Never expect a partner to perform fellatio if there is any infection present.

To perform fellatio, begin by kissing the shaft and then the tip of his penis. The underside of the glans – particularly around the frenulum – is the most sensitive part. The testicles are also sensitive to the lips and tongue. Despite the fact that giving oral sex to a man is sometimes known as a 'blow job' do NOT blow. Moisten his penis with the tongue and lick it as you would an ice cream. Then slip your lips around the glans of the penis and lower your head a little. Move your head up and down slowly and move your tongue around his penis.

FOUR POSITIONS FOR FELLATIO

1. He stands and she kneels in front of him.

2. He sits in a chair. She kneels in front of him and lowers her head into his lap.

3. He lies flat on his back and she kneels over him.

4. He kneels on the floor and sits back on his haunches. She lies on the floor in front of him with her face in his lap.

TO COME OR NOT TO COME

When performing fellatio for the first time most women worry about the same thing: 'Will he come in my mouth?' Ideally, this is something for couples to discuss together (though many are too embarrassed to discuss this). Whether or not he does come in your mouth is a question of taste – hers. And the same goes for whether or not to spit or swallow. Some women like the salty, bitter taste of semen. Others dislike it.

If you want him to come in your mouth and want to swallow but don't like the taste then you could experiment with a deep throat or deep mouth technique, taking his penis to the back of your mouth and allowing him to ejaculate straight into your stomach. This is a trick rather akin to sword-swallowing and takes a good deal of practice. If you want him to come in your mouth but don't want to swallow then you should have a handkerchief ready, as rushing out to the bathroom immediately may spoil the atmosphere. He should try to warn you before-hand when he is near the point of ejaculation.

If you don't want him to come in your mouth, then he should respect your wish and make sure that he pulls out of your mouth in time. Some women who do not like their partners to ejaculate in their mouths like to watch their partners orgasm and may like to catch the semen in their hands or on their breasts. The important thing is to discuss this beforehand.

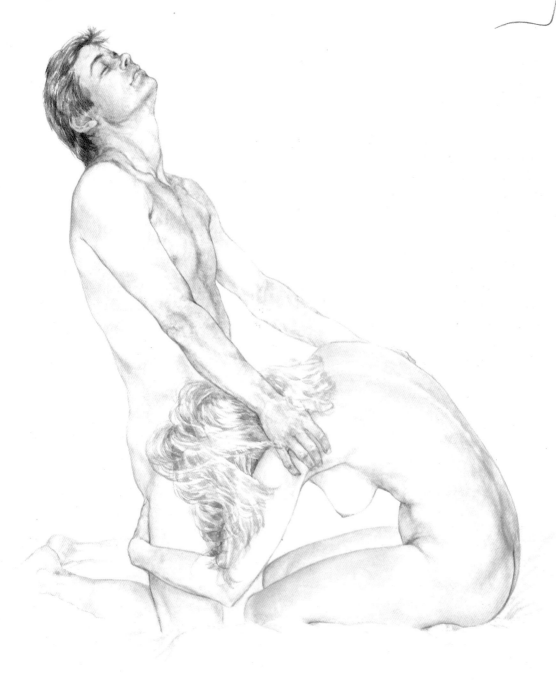

MASTURBATION

Most people begin their sex lives by learning how to masturbate. It used to be thought that masturbation was an exclusively male habit but it isn't. Women do it too. And no one need be afraid of long-term consequences. No one ever went blind (or even short-sighted) as a result of masturbating!

There are many times when it will be appropriate for one partner to masturbate the other to an orgasm. If a woman has failed to orgasm during intercourse, for example, then her partner may help her reach an orgasm by masturbating her. Remember that MOST women do not usually reach an orgasm through sexual intercourse and do need to masturbate (or to be masturbated) to be sexually satisfied.

Many men and women feel shy or embarrassed about masturbation. Try not to allow your feelings to inhibit you. Talk to one another and show your partner what you would like them to do by moving their fingers a little in this direction and then a little in that direction; if you want them to press harder, don't be afraid of showing them what you want.

NOTES FOR HIM MASTURBATING HER

Don't just head straight for the clitoris. Be slow and gentle. Touch her mons veneris and the outer part of her vagina first. Move your fingers up and down, round and round and from side to side. Start with a whole hand massage and grad-ually concentrate on a smaller and smaller area (using fewer and fewer fingers) as you find out what she wants. Build up the speed and the pressure slowly. Try slipping a finger in between her vaginal lips. Press the ball of your hand just above her pubic bone. If she feels dry, dip your fingers in your mouth and moisten her with saliva. If your hands are rough use a baby oil or a plain hand cream. Make sure that your fingernails are cut short and that there are no ragged edges. Press one or more fingers into her vagina if that seems to give her any satisfaction. Gentle rubbing and pulling on the skin around the clitoris will probably produce just as good a result as touching the clitoris itself. With time you will get to know what she wants but if you are in any doubt ask her to show you (with her fingers) what will give her the most satisfaction.

NOTES FOR HER MASTURBATING HIM

Gently drag your nails along the skin of his scrotum and gently hold his scrotum in your fingers. Touch the skin between his scrotum and his anus. Run your fingers up and down the shaft of his penis. Hold his penis carefully between your fingers and move your fingers up and down. Ask him if he wants you to hold him tighter – or not so tightly. If you need a lubricant try saliva or baby oil. Speed up and slow down your movement to build up the suspense. If he has a foreskin move that up and down slowly. Either grip his penis with your thumb and first finger or with the whole of your hand. Don't be shy about watching when he ejaculates – he may find it an extra turn-on. Remember that when leaving the penis semen may travel several feet.

(No·No) ANAL SEX

Although anal sex is illegal in many parts of the world it is remarkably popular among heterosexuals. One in ten heterosexual couples regularly have anal sex and more than fifty per cent of heterosexuals have tried it.

NO INTEREST IN THIS

love this

1

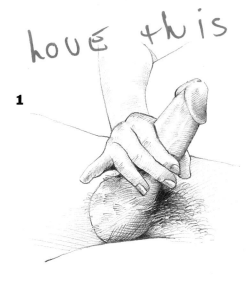

2

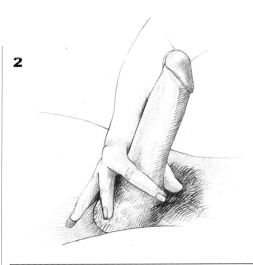

3

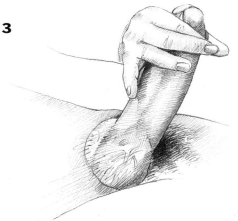

Anal sex first became popular as a means of avoiding conception. It is generally believed that the spread of AIDS in large parts of Africa can be partly explained by the fact that anal intercourse is still used for this purpose.

Today, however, most couples who practise anal sex do so because they find it more exciting. Men claim that penetrating a tight anal sphincter gives them a special type of pleasure, while women who like anal sex say that they get a more intense orgasm. Because anal sex is painful, it can appeal to men who like to be dominant and women who like to be submissive – though with the aid of a vibrator it is, of course, possible for a woman to take the dominant, assertive role. Anal sex is, in fact, the only way a woman can 'penetrate' a man.

If you want to try anal sex remember that lubrication is vital. There is little natural lubrication and the sphincter, which guards the rectum, is naturally very tight.

The 'active' partner should start by gently pushing a fingertip into the 'passive' partner's anus, pressing very gently. The 'passive' partner should bear down on the fingertip. It may help to tighten up the anal sphincter and then to let it relax. Once the sphincter is opened and well lubricated, penetration with a penis or vibrator can commence. The lubrication should be spread over the anus and the penis or vibrator. The anal sphincter normally closes automatically when any object approaches from outside, so the active partner will need a considerable amount of determination to overcome this natural barrier. The passive partner should try hard to relax. You are unlikely to be able to penetrate very far on your first attempts. With practice, it is possible for either or both partners to reach an orgasm in this position.

There are various sexual positions that are suitable for anal intercourse. Any of the rear entry positions will do, but the standard rear entry position is probably the most popular and the easiest to achieve.

VARIATIONS ON THE SEXUAL THEME

It is possible to have sex without using the vagina or the anus. If ordinary sex is impossible for any reason and you want to try an alternative to sex or masturbation here are some possibilities:

INTERMAMMILLARY SEX

If the woman's breasts are large enough to be squeezed together to make a channel, then intermammillary sex (sex between the breasts) may be possible. She can lie flat on her back and pull her breasts together over her chest. He then kneels over her and places his penis in between her breasts while she keeps squeezing her breasts together. If she wants to take a passive role, he can mould her breasts around his penis and use them as a masturbatory aid. Alternatively, she can kneel over him and hold her breasts around his penis and take control.

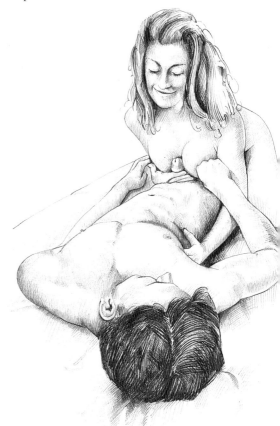

INTERFEMORAL SEX

This technique is widely used by transvestite male prostitutes. 'She' holds her thighs together tightly and he pushes his penis in between them. The standard rear entry positions are most suitable although it is possible to penetrate from the front – when, for example, 'she' is standing. She must keep her legs fairly tightly together.

GLUTEAL SEX

The crease between the mound of the buttocks can be used as a vaginal alternative. This position can be used with both partners standing and facing in the same direction. If she contracts her gluteal (buttock) muscles and rotates her pelvis while he thrusts, then he at least should be able to reach an orgasm.

FINDING THE RIGHT POSITION

Most couples have two or three favourite positions and even when they try new positions may return to their old, well-tried positions, either because they find that these positions provide most satisfaction or because they have happy memories of their sexual experiences in those positions. It is worth remembering that:

• Just because you start off having sex in one position it doesn't mean that you have to finish in the same position. Many couples change position several times while making love, first finding a position that she likes, then trying something that he likes.
• There is no such thing as a 'perfect' sexual position. Whatever gives you BOTH satisfaction is right for YOU.
• Different positions offer different types of pleasure, but not necessarily different degrees of pleasure.
• Past experiences – happy or unhappy – may lead to long lasting preferences for particular sexual positions.

• Battles outside the bedroom can lead to battles in the bedroom. If a couple are constantly fighting for dominance in their everyday relationship, then the fight will probably spill over into the bedroom, with potentially disastrous results.
• Long-standing attitudes towards sex may make it difficult for some individuals to try particular positions. For example, men who believe that a woman's place is underneath may find it difficult to make love in the 'woman on top' position. And women who have been brought up to believe that a woman should be submissive during sex may find it difficult to take an assertive role.
• You may be able to discover things about yourself, your partner and your relationship by analysing your favourite sexual position. If she always insists on taking the 'woman on top' position then she is probably striving to dominate the relationship. If he is only happy with the 'rear entry position' then he is probably aggressive and dominant and if he is unhappy with the 'woman on top' position then he is probably sensitive, or maybe insecure about his masculine role.

FACTORS WHICH INFLUENCE THE CHOICE OF POSITION

1. Physical deformities. If she suffers from backache or he has bad arthritis in his knees then there will be a natural, physical restriction on the available positions. There is no point at all in even trying a sexual position which is painful for one or both partners.

2. Weight. If one partner is much heavier than the other then both partners will probably be happier with a position in which the lighter partner is on top. For example, if the man is much heavier than the woman, then the missionary position will be less suitable than the woman on top positions. Remember that there are many variations on this position.

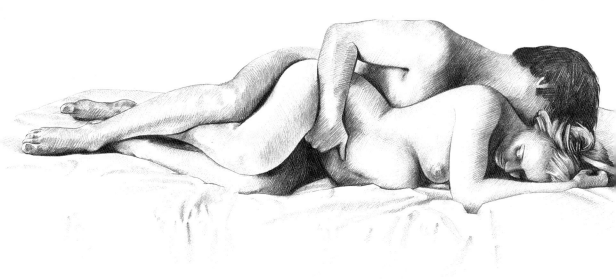

3. Pregnancy. Positions which put least strain on the woman's abdomen are advisable. Rear entry positions, side by side positions and woman on top positions are all much better than the missionary position for pregnant women.

4. Size of sexual organs. Positions in which deep penetration is inevitable will probably not be suitable if he has an unusually large penis and she has an unusually small vagina. On the other hand if she has an exceptionally spacious vagina and he has a particularly small penis then a deep penetration position will probably be useful.

5. Fears and hang ups. There is no point at all in choosing a position that appeals to one of you if the other is terrified or embarrassed. The golden rule is that you should never do – or even try – anything that both of you are not entirely happy about.

6. Her ability to reach an orgasm. If a woman has a great deal of difficulty in reaching an orgasm during normal intercourse then it is sensible either to choose a position in which the clitoris receives the greatest amount of natural stimulation, or to choose one in which it will be

possible for one or both partners to manually stimulate the clitoris during intercourse.

7. His ability to maintain a firm erection. Some positions need a really firm erection – others can be managed successfully with an erection that is only moderately firm.

8. Her need to dominate. Some women are only really satisfied by a sexual position in which they can take an assertive, dominating role. Such women usually prefer woman on top positions – and usually prefer to remain active during sex, rather than passive.

9. His need to dominate. Some men feel uncomfortable if they are not in a dominating and assertive position during sex.

10. Her need to be dominated. Some women only feel comfortable during sex if they know that their partner is in charge.

11. His need to be dominated. Less commonly, some men feel more comfortable when the woman they are making love to is assertive and takes charge.

12. A desire to find a position in which both partners can see what is happening. Some people are turned on by being able to see what is going on – in other words to see their sexual organs in action.

13. A desire to be able to kiss. Some people feel uncomfortable if they cannot kiss during sex. Without kissing they feel that sex becomes too impersonal, clinical and lacking in emotional intimacy.

14. A desire to see one another's bodies. In some positions the two partners face in opposite directions. Visual contact disappears completely. Some men and women strongly dislike this type of sex and prefer to be able to see one another.

15. His desire to touch her breasts. Men are often stimulated sexually by being able to touch their partner's breasts.

16. A desire for maximum skin contact. Many people like to be in touch with their partner's bodies during sex. Skin contact makes sex more intimate and more enjoyable.

17. A desire to share everything. Some couples prefer positions in which all aspects of the physical relationship can be shared with no one partner dominant.

18. Her need to touch her clitoris. Because many women can only reach orgasm if they masturbate or are masturbated, positions in which the woman can touch her own clitoris are often popular.

19. A need for contact that is exclusively genital. There are some positions in which contact is (almost) exclusively genital.

20. A desire for prolonged intercourse. If he suffers from premature ejaculation – or both partners want their love-making to last longer – then they may want to experiment with a variety of sexual positions in which their orgasms are likely to be delayed and intercourse is prolonged.

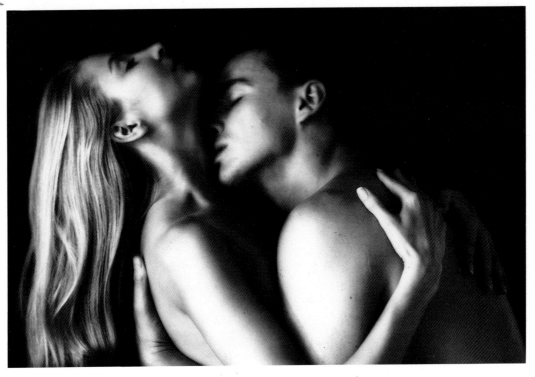

CHOOSING THE IDEAL POSITION FOR YOU –

Some Suggestions (see code below)

1. Want close skin contact
M, M1, M3, W2, W5, W9, R1, R8, S

2. Both want to watch sex organs in action
W, W3, W5, W9

3. He wants to be able to touch her breasts
M1, M3, M7, W, W9, R2, R10

4. She wants to be able to masturbate herself
M4, M6, W, W1, W9, R8

5. Main contact is genital
M6, R3

6. Want to prolong intercourse
W, W1, W2, W3, W4, W5, W6, W7

7. She is pregnant
R10, S

8. He is much heavier than her
W, W1, W8, R10

9. She is much heavier than him
M, M1, R10

10. Both want to be able to see one another
M, M1, M3, W5

11. Want to be able to kiss
M, M1, M3, W2, W9

12. Problems with a firm erection
R10

13. She wants a position where her clitoris will receive maximum stimulation
M1, M3, W, W1

14. Want a position for a quick getaway
M7, R7, R8

15. He has an unusually large penis
W, W1, W2, W3, W4, W5, W6, W8, R3, R5, R8

16. He has an unusually small penis
M2, M4, R, R3, R4, R6, R9

17. She wants to dominate
W, W1, W2, W3, W4, W5, W6, W7, W8, R8

18. He wants to dominate
M, M1, M2, M3, M4, R, R1, R2, R6, R7

19. No one dominates
R5, S

20. They want a position where deep penetration is possible
M2, M4, R, R2, R5, R6, R9

CODE

M =	basic missionary position
M1 =	missionary variation 1
M2 =	missionary variation 2
M3 =	missionary variation 3
M4 =	missionary variation 4
M5 =	missionary variation 5
M6 =	missionary variation 6
M7 =	missionary variation 7
W =	basic woman on top position
W1 =	woman on top variation 1
W2 =	woman on top variation 2
W3 =	woman on top variation 3
W4 =	woman on top variation 4
W5 =	woman on top variation 5
W6 =	woman on top variation 6
W7 =	woman on top variation 7
W8 =	woman on top variation 8
W9 =	woman on top variation 9
R =	basic rear entry position
R1 =	rear entry variation 1
R2 =	rear entry variation 2
R3 =	rear entry variation 3
R4 =	rear entry variation 4
R5 =	rear entry variation 5
R6 =	rear entry variation 6
R7 =	rear entry variation 7
R8 =	rear entry variation 8
R9 =	rear entry variation 9
R10 =	rear entry variation 10
S =	basic side by side position

AFTERPLAY

When a man has ejaculated his interest in sex (and his partner) may decline rapidly. As his penis shrinks so does his sex drive. Many men fall asleep as soon as they have had an orgasm. This is a physiological consequence of sex rather than a comment or an insult. Human sexual urges were designed for procreation and when a man has ejaculated his purpose is done: if he remains sexually interested he will be more likely to hinder than to help the process of conception.

Women are quite different. They remain alert, sensitive and loving after intercourse. Many say that their need for love and reassurance and comfort is greater after sex than at any other time. They are likely to feel lonely, abandoned, depressed and used if their partner rolls over and falls asleep the minute he has ejaculated, especially if she has not had an orgasm or has not been sexually satisfied.

This problem can to a certain extent be alleviated by making love in the morning when you are both wide awake rather than at night when you are both tired (and he is, therefore, more likely to fall asleep anyway).

And women should remember that men are more vulnerable and more sensitive than they appear to be. Rushing off to the bathroom after making love will not do his ego much good. Keep a towel or box of tissues nearby if you want to avoid the inevitable damp patch on the sheets. And be careful not to say anything that could be construed as critical. If you want to talk, avoid household problems and concentrate on romantic plans and aspirations for the future.

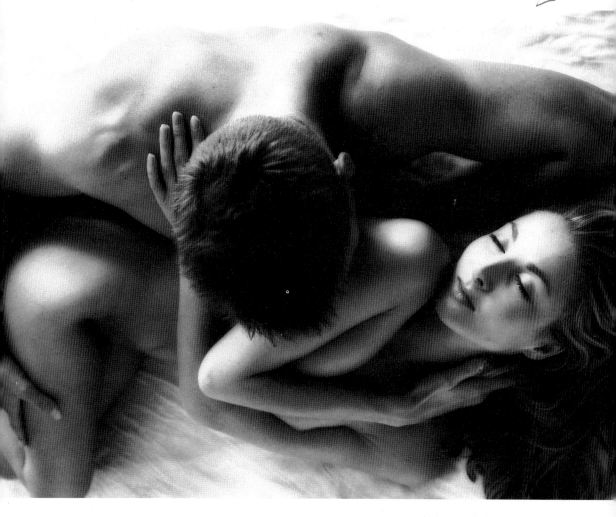

CHAPTER FOUR

Male Sexual Problems

Impotence and premature ejaculation are the two most common sexual problems to affect men. Both problems cause an enormous amount of anxiety.

IMPOTENCE

Impotence always seems to be the end of the world to a previously virile male. It usually strikes at the most inopportune and embarrassing moment. It certainly strikes at the moment when a man is at his most vulnerable.

Most, probably all men, are impotent at one time or another. The symptoms are simple: he cannot acquire an erection easily and/or if he does get one then it is either too weak or too short-lived to enable him to penetrate his partner.

Here are some of the most likely causes. As you will see most are not serious.

FEAR

Many types of fear can produce impotence. A man will have difficulty in acquiring an erection if he is frightened of catching a disease, of being caught, of making his partner pregnant, of hurting her or causing himself pain.

TIREDNESS

Tiredness, often through overwork, is a common cause of impotence and it is quite normal to have difficulty in acquiring or maintaining an erection when tired.

INADEQUACY

Some men feel very inadequate about their bodies, not simply about the size or shape of their penises. Some men cannot comfortably make love to women whom they consider to be beautiful; they may often feel happier with a woman who they consider very plain, who takes no pride in herself or even a woman who is deformed. Prostitutes who are blind, have amputated limbs or severe, disabling disorders often do surprisingly well.

ANXIETY

Anxiety about failure is a common cause of impotence. The risk of failure is proportional to the build-up. If a man really wants to impress his partner then the chances of him being impotent are high. Men who worry about how well they are doing are also prone to impotence. A man who is making love to a woman he really loves (or fancies) for the first time will often discover that he is impotent; his desire to do well will be too much for him.

OBESITY

Men who are fat are more likely to suffer from impotence. (Note: sexual positions in which the woman is on top are most suitable for men who are severely overweight.)

ALCOHOL

A modest amount of alcohol will increase the desire for sex but too much will adversely affect performance. Most 'leisure' drugs (from tobacco to heroin) can cause problems. Smoking is a major cause of impotence.

DISEASE

Diseases such as diabetes can cause impotence.

GUILT

A man who tries to make love to a woman other than his wife will be prone to impotence.

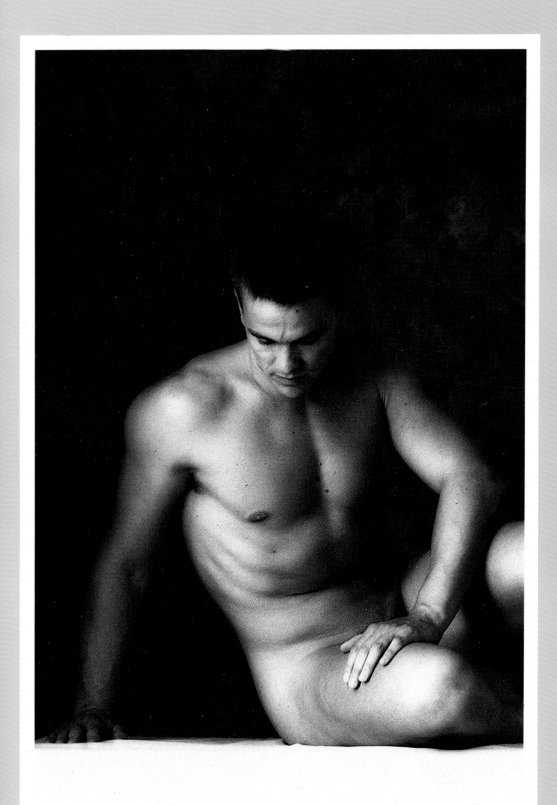

MEMORIES

A man who tries to make love in a room or bed he associates with someone else may suffer from impotence, as may a man who tries to make love to a woman who has been a friend or a former partner of a friend for many years.

DRUGS

Prescribed drugs – particularly drugs which are used in the treatment of high blood pressure or depression can cause impotence.

OVERCOMING IMPOTENCE

If you are suffering from impotence, you must slowly and gradually rebuild your confidence. You should try to deal with any anxieties or problems in other parts of your life and spend a little time learning how to relax. You will find it easier to conquer your impotence if you have one regular partner rather than a number of occasional partners or a succession of one night stands. With new partners you will have to explain your problem repeatedly and will undoubtedly find it more stressful.

Spend time on foreplay. Learn how to please your partner in ways other than full intercourse. If you know that you can bring your partner to orgasm before you have entered her then the pressure on you will be reduced enormously. Try to relax with your partner as often as you can – and to cuddle and kiss frequently.

Some experts recommend that men who are suffering from impotence should make a decision to try not to have intercourse for six weeks. During that time you should just touch your partner. You should become adept at foreplay. Even if you have an erection you should not have sex. You should learn to relax and enjoy your partner. Bring her to orgasm with your hands and encourage her to do the same for you.

If, after six weeks, you are regularly getting erections then you can make love. If not then you should extend your period of deliberate abstinence for another four weeks. Taking the pressure off in this way can work wonders.

THESE ARE SOME TIPS FOR ANY MAN SUFFERING FROM IMPOTENCE.

1. THE FIRST AND MOST IMPORTANT THING TO REMEMBER IS THAT IMPOTENCE PROBABLY AFFECTS EVERY MAN IN THE WORLD AT ONE TIME OR ANOTHER. IF YOU DO OCCASIONALLY GET AN ERECTION (ASLEEP OR AWAKE, ALONE OR WITH A PARTNER) THEN THERE IS NOTHING PHYSICALLY WRONG WITH YOUR EQUIPMENT. THE PROBLEM IS IN YOUR MIND AND CAN BE CONQUERED. THE VAST MAJORITY OF CASES OF IMPOTENCE FIT INTO THIS CATEGORY.

2. THE MORE YOU WORRY ABOUT THE PROBLEM THE WORSE IT IS LIKELY TO GET.

3. IF YOU ARE TOTALLY UNABLE TO HAVE AN ERECTION AT ANY TIME THEN YOUR PROBLEM MAY NEED TREATMENT WITH HORMONES. TALK TO YOUR DOCTOR.

4. DO NOT WASTE YOUR MONEY ON 'QUACK' REMEDIES. WAY BACK IN THE EIGHTEENTH CENTURY IN ITALY IMPOTENT MEN PRESENTED THEIR SLUGGISH AND RELUCTANT ORGANS TO SAINT DAMIEN AND BEGGED FOR HIS HELP. TODAY MEN ARE MORE LIKELY TO PAY FOR WEIRD CONCOCTIONS ORDERED FROM THE SMALL ADS. BECAUSE OF THE SHAME AND EMBARRASSMENT THAT THEY FEEL IMPOTENT MEN OFTEN DARE NOT COMPLAIN WHEN THE PRODUCT TURNS OUT TO BE WORTHLESS.

Finally, if your erection is a poor one you will find that penetration is far easier to achieve if you lie side by side or with the women on top. The missionary position is not good for men who suffer from partial impotence.

CASE HISTORY: JOHN'S NIGHTMARE

John's nightmare came true one Friday evening.

John is single and unattached and for weeks he had fancied a girl he worked with: Diane was tall, blonde, 27 years old, curvy and vivacious.

It took John ages to pluck up the courage to ask Diane out. He asked around the office first and confirmed that she was single and unattached. He couldn't believe it and still didn't have the courage to ask her for a date.

Eventually, at the beginning of one week, he took the plunge and asked her to go to the cinema with him. To his intense delight, she agreed. He was a nervous wreck all week. He had been dreaming of her for ages and could hardly believe that she wanted to go out with him.

They went for a meal and then to the cinema and got on wonderfully well. John could feel the envious eyes of just about every man around fixed on him and his date.

After the film had finished they went dancing in a local nightclub. It was John's first chance to get physically close to her. He held her, kissed her and felt the hair on the back of his neck stand up with the excitement. And then they went back to John's flat together.

That is when the nightmare started.

'It's never happened before,' John said. 'But I just couldn't get an erection. It was terrible – I was totally impotent.'

He said that it wasn't the drink – he'd had hardly anything alcoholic because he'd been driving. And it certainly wasn't Diane; he'd never in his life fancied anyone as much as he had fancied her. And it wasn't that she was unwilling – he said that it was Diane who made the first move when they got back to his flat.

'The worst thing was,' said John afterwards, 'that as soon as Diane had gone home, I developed the biggest and firmest erection I have ever had in my life.' The only possible explanation is that John was simply suffering from anxiety. He really liked Diane, he wanted to impress her and he was too anxious for the evening to go well.

The risk of failure is always proportional to the amount of anxiety and the determination of a man to prove himself a great lover. Any man who is making love to a woman he really likes for the first time will be likely to discover that he is impotent – his desire to do well will often be too much for him.

John's best move now is to try to explain all this to Diane, to try to arrange another date and to rebuild his confidence slowly and steadily. If Diane fancies him just half as much as he fancies her then there shouldn't be any real problem, and she may even be flattered to know just how great an effect she had on him.

PREMATURE EJACULATION

Some experts argue that any ejaculation which happens before both partners are ready for it is, in fact, premature. Other groups argue that a man is a premature ejaculator if he cannot withhold ejaculation long enough for his partner to have an orgasm fifty per cent of the time; or if he cannot stop himself ejaculating for at least a minute after entering his partner; or if he ejaculates before he can get his penis into his partner's vagina.

Premature ejaculation occurs mainly in younger men and tends to disappear after the age of thirty when the reflexes become duller. It is so common that at least one-half of all men ejaculate too quickly the first time they make love to an attractive new partner (though the second attempt is usually much more successful).

Premature ejaculation is primarily a psychological problem rather than a physical one. It is commonly caused by over-enthusiasm, great expectations, excitement and anxiety. Over-eagerness to please is probably the most common cause, and anxiety about it happening is almost certain to make it worse.

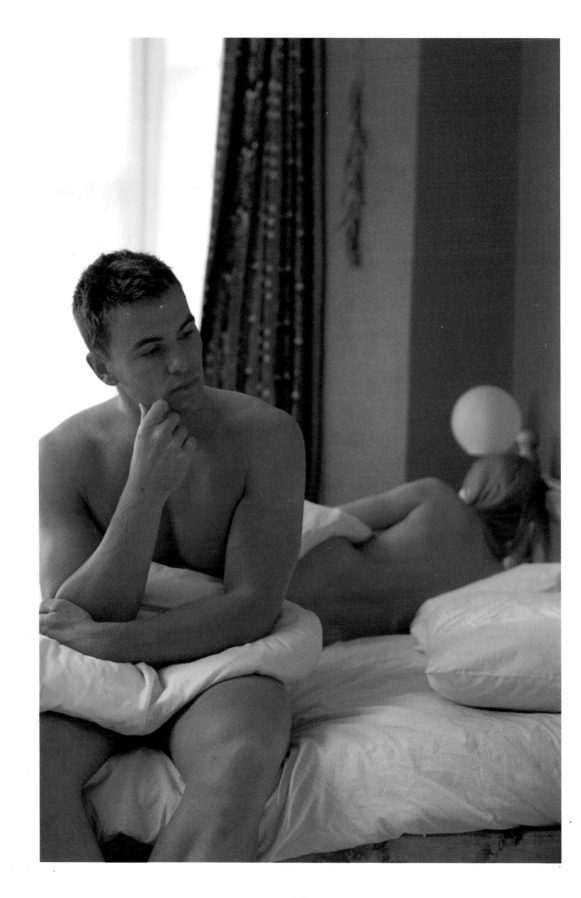

TIPS FOR MEN WHO WANT TO CONQUER PREMATURE EJACULATION

1. Try wearing a condom during intercourse. The condom will help to reduce the stimulation that hastens an orgasm.

2. Try using a local anaesthetic cream, available from any good pharmacy. The cream will have the same 'dulling' effect as wearing a condom and therefore should help to prolong your erection.

3. Most men find that their second erection disappears much less speedily than their first. So, if the first ends quickly in a premature ejaculation, and disappointment for both partners, wait a while and then try again.

4. It is sometimes possible to extend the lifespan of an erection by distracting yourself with some sexually unstimulating thought. Some men actually attempt to do mathematical problems or try to work out their difficulties at work while making love in order to prolong the life of an erection.

5. Tense your buttock muscles while making love: this should help you to delay the moment of orgasm.

6. Satisfy your partner orally or manually before you enter her. Knowing that she will not be left frustrated – however quickly you ejaculate – should help reduce the pressure and enable you to last far longer.

7. Gently pull down your testicles before penetration and during intercourse. Prior to ejaculation the testicles normally rise slowly towards the base of the penis. By pulling them (very gently) in the opposite direction you may be able to delay orgasm.

8. Many young men learn to come quickly, possibly because they are frightened of being discovered while masturbating. You may be able to teach yourself to come more slowly by trying to delay your orgasm as long as possible while masturbating.

9. Recruit your partner's help. She should sit on the bed with her back resting against the bed-head. You lie near to her so that she can hold your penis in her hand. She then masturbates you. The moment you feel that you are about to ejaculate you should tell her. She should then gently squeeze your penis at the point where the glans meets the shaft, holding it still for around five seconds. This should arrest the ejaculation. Both relax for a minute or so before she resumes

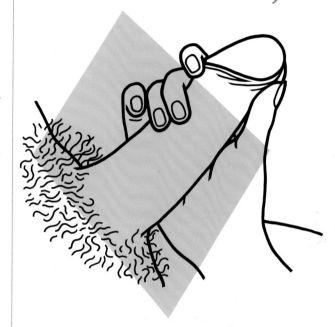

masturbating you. Using this technique should enable you gradually to build up your resistance – and your confidence in your resistance. Your partner can use a lubricant on her hand to simulate conditions inside her vagina. Once you are satisfied that you are making good progress with this technique you can begin practising inside your partner's vagina.

She should take the woman on top position and you should keep quite still. She then moves, slowly and carefully, and you tell her if you feel that you are close to coming. She should then keep still for a few moments until you feel that it is safe for her to continue. After practising this technique for a while most men notice a considerable improvement in their ability to dealy ejaculation. It is, of course, vital to have a sympathetic and patient partner.

FACTS ABOUT PREMATURE EJACULATION

1. WHEN MAN LIVED IN THE WILD PREMATURE EJACULATION WAS SOMETHING OF AN ASSET. IN THE DAYS WHEN MEN WERE EATEN ALIVE BY WILD ANIMALS, A MAN WHO TOOK A LONG TIME OVER SEX MIGHT FIND HIMSELF BEING EATEN BEFORE HE COULD PROCREATE. A MAN WHO TOOK TOO LONG TO EJACULATE PROBABLY DIDN'T FATHER TOO MANY CHILDREN.

2. IT IS MORE COMMON AMONG MEN WHO DO NOT HAVE SEX VERY OFTEN AND, PARADOXICALLY PERHAPS, AMONG MEN WHO MASTURBATE A GREAT DEAL.

3. IT IS SOMETIMES SAID THAT WHEREAS A MEAT DIET TENDS TO INCREASE A MAN'S CHANCES OF BECOMING A PREMATURE EJACULATOR, A VEGETARIAN DIET MAKES IT MUCH LESS LIKELY.

4. MEN SOMETIMES EJACULATE PREMATURELY IF THEY FEEL THAT THEIR PARTNER REGARDS SEX AS AN UNWELCOME IMPOSITION.

5. SOMETIMES MEN WHOSE PARTNERS HAVE JUST GIVEN BIRTH WILL EJACULATE PREMATURELY. PSYCHOLOGISTS ARGUE THAT THEY FEEL BAD ABOUT HAVING SEX WITH A WOMAN WHO IS A MOTHER AND SO (DRIVEN BY A SUBCONSCIOUS FORCE) TRY TO GET IT OVER WITH AS QUICKLY AS POSSIBLE.

6. MEN WHO WERE STARVED OF AFFECTION AND LOVE WHEN YOUNG ARE OFTEN PREMATURE EJACULATORS.

7. SOME WOMEN FEAR THAT IF THEIR PARTNER EJACULATES PREMATURELY IT MUST BE BECAUSE HE DOESN'T 'FANCY' THEM, OR BECAUSE HE IS THINKING ABOUT SOME OTHER WOMAN. BOTH THEORIES ARE WRONG.

8. MANY MEN WHO WORRY THAT THEY ARE EJACULATING PREMATURELY IN FACT LAST BETWEEN ONE AND SIX MINUTES AFTER PENETRATION. THIS IS WITHIN NORMAL LIMITS. IT IS RARE FOR A MAN TO BE ABLE TO LAST FOR THE TEN MINUTES OR SO THAT THE AVERAGE WOMAN NEEDS TO REACH AN ORGASM.

MOST WOMEN WHO DO REACH ORGASM DIRECTLY AND SOLELY THROUGH INTERCOURSE NEED AT LEAST TEN MINUTES OF SOLID, HARD THRUSTING. THAT SORT OF REQUIREMENT CAN MAKE SEX FAR TOO MUCH LIKE HARD WORK FOR MANY MEN. IT IS PROBABLY BETTER FOR BOTH PARTNERS TO ACCEPT THAT SHE IS UNLIKELY TO REACH ORGASM THROUGH INTERCOURSE ALONE AND BETTER IF HE HELPS HER REACH ORGASM THROUGH MANUAL OR ORAL CLITORAL STIMULATION, OR IF SHE HELPS HERSELF TO AN ORGASM THROUGH MASTURBATION.

Robert has suffered from premature ejaculation for a year – and he believes it has stopped him from developing a proper relationship with a woman.

During the last twelve months he has tried to make love to five different women. And each time he has tried, it has been a dismal and embarrassing failure. On each sad occasion he has ejaculated within a couple of seconds of starting to make love.

'I'm doomed to one night stands,' he complained. 'I never have the courage to ring a woman up after I've failed so abysmally. So I have to move on to another relationship and try again.'

For months Robert refused to seek help. He was too embarrassed to tell anyone about his problem. He had wasted a considerable amount of money on purchaseing special vitamin and mineral supplements which would, according to the advertisements he saw, solve his problem speedily and permanently.

What Robert did not realize was that it is extremely common for a man to suffer from premature ejaculation when making love to a new partner for the first time, especially when he is nervous or too anxious about his performance.

Robert is most likely to be able to solve his problem permanently if he makes an effort to build up a relationship with one woman – and he will be particularly likely to succeed if he can find the courage to talk to his partner about the problem and, ideally, to enlist her help. Premature ejaculation is far less likely to affect a man who has one regular partner, than it is a man who tries to make love to an endless series of comparative strangers.

> *"What Robert did not realize was that it is extremely common for a man to suffer from premature ejaculation."*

PRIAPISM

Priapism is a disorder named after a Roman god who had a large, stiff wooden penis; it is a condition in which a man has a permanent erection. It is an erection he doesn't want, gets no sexual pleasure out of and cannot get rid of. Erections of this type occur for several reasons. They can happen during the night or develop after taking a prescribed drug. Anyone who suffers from priapism should consult their doctor as soon as possible for specialist medical help.

RETARDED EJACULATION

Retarded ejaculation is the opposite to premature ejaculation –but it happens much less often. Men may have difficulty in reaching orgasm for a number of reasons:

1. They have deliberately tried to hold back (either in the hope that their partner will reach her orgasm or in an attempt to avoid the risk of making their partner pregnant). Afterwards, when they then try to ejaculate they find that they can no longer come and that they have 'gone past the point of no return'.

2. They feel guilty about ejaculating. If a man is worried for any reason (he may be making love to a woman who is not his wife or he may be worried about pregnancy) then he may have difficulty in obtaining an erection or, if he does have an erection, he may have difficulty in ejaculating.

3. They may have drunk too much alcohol or taken too many reflex dulling pills.

Men who suffer from retarded ejaculation can sometimes help themselves by using their imagination, by persuading their partner to try a different position, or by masturbating to a position close to orgasm and then continuing with normal sexual intercourse. Sometimes the female partner may be able to help by using a different technique, by providing manual stimulation or by initiating fellatio. Communication between partners is vital.

CHAPTER FIVE

Female Sexual Problems

Like men, women are vulnerable to psychological problems such as guilt and anxiety. However, some of the sexual problems that afflict them are caused by hormonal changes or by infections, which may require medical advice and treatment.

VAGINISMUS

The majority of women who have never had sex before are nervous and apprehensive. When they see an erect penis for the first time they wonder how on earth it is going to fit inside them: they have no idea just how capacious the female vagina can become. Things may be made worse by the fact that they have been led to believe that their first sexual experience will be painful.

Normally, the vagina is extremely flexible. However narrow it may seem to be, it can quickly and readily expand to cope with the thickest penis. But if the muscles around the vagina are tense, the vagina will not expand and with those vaginal muscles tightly contracted, penetration will be so painful as to be impossible. This condition – known as vaginismus – is widely regarded as the female equivalent of impotence.

When the male partner tries to insert his penis into the 'nervous' vagina he invariably makes things worse. The more he pushes the more the muscles contract and the more impossible the task becomes. The anxiety creates muscle spasm, the muscle spasm makes penetration painful and the pain creates more anxiety. What probably started out as a slight discomfort soon becomes a severe and raging pain, and vaginal muscle spasms soon ensure that the penis does not enter the vagina.

Sometimes the fear of pain – and the very real pain that can develop – is only part of the story. Cultural, religious and parental pressures may conspire to persuade a woman that what she is doing is wrong. These feelings are particularly likely to develop if, for any reason, the woman harbours any feeling of guilt (which may not be obvious) about the sexual relationship.

It is worth remembering at this point that although vaginismus in virgins is usually psychological there *can* be physical causes. Any virgin who finds sexual intercourse painful or impossible should ask her own doctor for a check up to make sure, for example, that there is no unbroken hymen (see page 77).

Although vaginismus is a condition which most commonly affects virgins, it can affect women who are sexually experienced. When this happens there can be several reasons.

First, there are the physical causes.

• An infection may make intercourse painful.

• Hormonal changes (such as those which take place during the menopause) may mean that there is relatively little lubrication inside the vagina, making penetration painful.

• A scar may have developed after a woman has had a baby. Or if a woman suffered a tear after giving birth, the repair may have been done clumsily so that there is genuinely insufficient room left for a penis to enter. (Sometimes, after giving birth, a woman who has had a number of babies, and who has an unusually lax vagina may encourage the surgeon performing the repair to 'tighten things up a bit'. The surgeon's over-

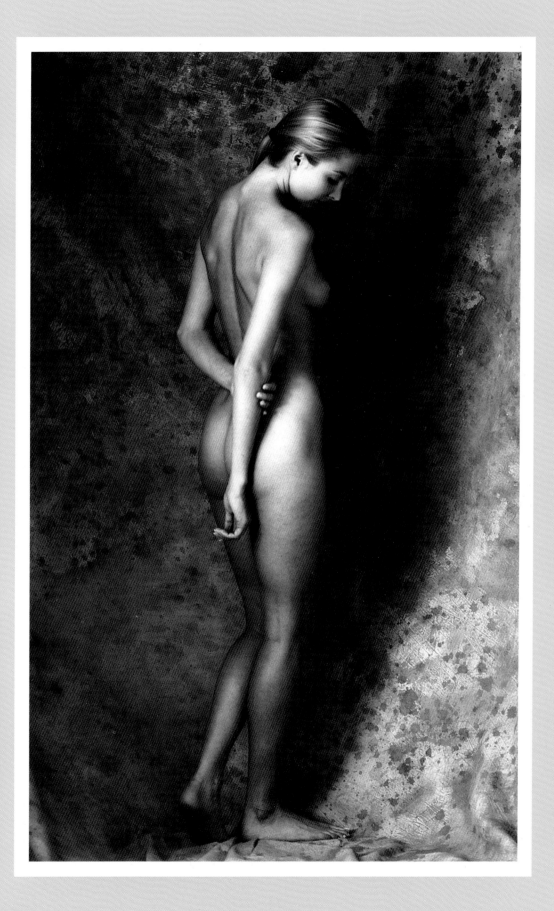

enthusiastic interpretation of her request may lead to problems). To make sure that there are no physical causes for vaginismus, it is wise to seek a medical opinion.

Second, there are the psychological causes of vaginismus in sexually experienced women:

- **A MARRIED WOMAN WHO IS HAVING SEX WITH A NEW LOVER MAY FEEL GUILTY, AND HER GUILT MAY TURN INTO VAGINAL MUSCLE SPASM. IT IS NOT AT ALL UNCOMMON FOR A WOMAN TO BE RELAXED AND PERFECTLY CAPABLE OF SEX WITH ONE PARTNER BUT TO BE TENSE AND TIGHT WITH ANOTHER. STRANGELY, PERHAPS, A WOMAN MAY BE PERFECTLY CAPABLE OF HAVING SEX WITH HER LOVER BUT QUITE INCAPABLE OF HAVING SEX WITH HER HUSBAND!**

- **A SEXUALLY EXPERIENCED WOMAN WHO IS ANXIOUS TO PLEASE HER LOVER MAY BE SO TENSE AND NERVOUS THAT HER VAGINAL MUSCLES GO INTO SPASM AND CANNOT EASILY BE RELAXED.**

There are two relatively simple things that any woman can do to rebuild her confidence and to conquer her problem.

The first thing she should do is to take the pressure off herself by agreeing (with her partner) not to try to make love for six weeks or so. Both partners should cuddle and touch one another and, if the relationship is a new one, try to get used to being naked with one another. She should get used to looking at and touching his penis. Mutual masturbation is an excellent way to get rid of some initial fears and anxieties while finding some immediate short-term satisfaction. The important thing is that the process should not be rushed. The more nervous she is the more slowly and gently she should take things.

Next, she should gradually get used to the idea of having something inside her vagina by following these steps:

1. Make sure that you will not be disturbed and undress. It is a good idea to make sure that the room is warm since you will find it nigh on impossible to relax properly in a cold room.

2. Lie down flat on your back on your bed and raise your knees up so that your feet are flat on the bed. Put a pillow under your bottom to improve the angle of approach.

3. Wet the tip of your index finger with a little saliva.

4. Very, very gently push the tip of your finger in between your labia and into your vagina. Be very gentle. There is no need to hurry. If it hurts, stop. And stop when you are convinced that you cannot get your finger any further inside.

5. Continue this exercise the following day – but try to get your finger a little further inside.

6. Repeat the exercise every day until you can get your finger right inside you. Remember to wet it each time with saliva. If you prefer you can use a little baby oil.

7. Once you are happy that you can get a finger inside your vagina try with a tampon. Take the tampon out of its cardboard applicator and smear the end with baby oil or saliva. Then slowly push the tampon into your vagina in exactly the same way that you pushed your finger inside.

8. Once you can do this fairly easily and comfortably, try deliberately tightening up your vaginal muscles BEFORE you push the tampon inside yourself. Make your vaginal muscles as tight as you can and then put the tampon up against the entrance to your vagina. You will probably find that you cannot get the tampon inside. You'll probably find that you can't even get a finger inside. Now, deliberately relax the muscles that you have tightened. And as you do so bear down as though you were trying to push something out of your vagina. This movement will help you to relax and open up your vaginal muscles. While you are relaxing deliberately push the tampon into your vagina.

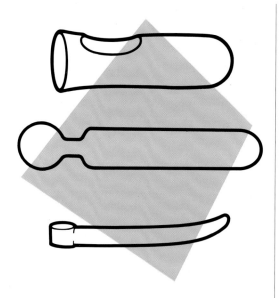

Dilators of varying thicknesses help women relax their vaginal muscles

9. At this stage most experts recommend that you start using proper vaginal dilators. These are usually made of glass and look rather like test-tubes (though they are solid). A set will consist of very thin dilators and quite thick ones. You should be able to borrow a set through your own doctor or gynaecologist. You use the dilators in exactly the same way as you used the tampon, starting with the thinnest and working your way up to the thickest. If you cannot get hold of a set of graduated dilators try using your fingers. Instead of using just one finger try using two. When you can get two fingers into your vagina without any pain or discomfort, try using three.

10. Once you have more confidence you can ask your partner to help you. Instead of using your own fingers or vaginal dilators try allowing him to put his finger(s) inside you. Remember that you are still in charge – you decide how many fingers are used and how far they go in. Do also remember that lubrication is vital and that if you haven't got anything else saliva is both safe and effective (assuming, of course, that you have no oral infection). Some male partners may be willing to prepare the vagina by applying the saliva direct from their own mouths.

11. Once the six week rest period is over – and as long as you are happy that your vagina can now accommodate at least two fingers at a time – you can try intercourse again. Don't rush. If you think you need longer then wait. Try to get yourself as relaxed as possible before trying. Make sure that the room is warm and that you use plenty of lubricant. And take things slowly. If sex is still impossible don't worry. You probably still need more practice. As with most sexual problems the really important thing is to be patient – and to have a patient and understanding partner.

CASE HISTORY: MANDY FOUND SEX TOO PAINFUL TO ENJOY

Only a true masochist enjoys sex which is painful - and there aren't many of them around. Mandy certainly wasn't a masochist but she hadn't enjoyed sex for several months when I first saw her.

There are a number of reasons why sex may hurt. Most aren't caused by serious problems.

Cuts, sores, localised infections, a lack of sufficient lubrication or an allergy reaction to a drug or cream of some sort can all cause superficial pains and soreness. Forgotten tampons inside the vagina can produce pain on intercourse, as can cystitis, an infection and inflammation of the bladder and urinary tract. A rigid hymen or a clumsy repair after a tear produced during childbirth can both cause pain. A deeper pain can be caused by endometriosis, fibroids, chronic pelvic congestion (a disorder which can be caused by repeatedly having intercourse without ever having an orgasm), ovarian cysts, a retroverted uterus or a prolapse.

I examined Mandy but could find no physical explanation for her complaint. And so we sat and talked, and eventually I began to understand why Mandy found sex too painful to enjoy.

Mandy, I discovered, was suffering from a condition known as vaginismus, an extremely common problem and one that many sex experts regard as the female equivalent of impotence.

Normally, the vagina is a very flexible tube. However narrow it may seem to be it is capable of expanding to accommodate even the thickest penis.

But sometimes the vagina does not expand; the vaginal muscles remain tightly contracted and attempts at penetration are simply too painful.

Most women who have never had sex before are nervous. They may actually expect sex to be painful, either because of something they have read or because of something they have been told, and so they involuntarily tighten up their muscles. When their partner tries to enter them they feel some initial discomfort and then they tighten up even more. The anxiety creates more pain and the pain reinforces the anxiety. Vaginal muscle spasms effectively keep the penis out of the vagina.

Mandy, however, was not a virgin and her vaginismus could not be explained so simply.

Guilt is a common cause of sexual problems in women. And it turned out that it was guilt that was causing Mandy's problem.

Any woman who is having sex with a new lover may feel guilty. If she is married and beginning an affair a woman may suffer enormous guilt, even though superficially she may be happy about what she is doing. It is not at all uncommon for a woman to suffer from vaginismus when she is with one sexual partner and to be relaxed and comfortable when she is with another.

I discovered that Mandy was getting divorced and had just begun a new relationship. She was still confused, bewildered and depressed about the breakdown of her old relationship, and when I talked to her it became clear that she was not yet ready for a new sexual relationship.

I advised Mandy to take the pressure off herself. I suggested that she and her lover should agree not to try to make love for another six weeks. They could, I told her, cuddle, touch one another, and get used to one anothers bodies but they should not attempt to have sex at all.

Mandy was able to talk to her new would-be lover easily and comfortably. He was sympathetic and reassuring, and told her that there was no hurry and no pressure. Time and good communication solved Mandy's problem far more effectively than any medical treatment could have done.

INABILITY TO HAVE AN ORGASM

It is a myth that every woman should be able to have an orgasm every time she has sex. This myth probably causes more heartache than any other. It is supplemented by the modern myth that every woman is entitled to a sequence of orgasms (a multiple orgasm) every time she has sexual intercourse.

The truth is that the majority of women do not normally have an orgasm during intercourse. Many women never have an orgasm during ordinary sexual intercourse. Most women only reach orgasm when they masturbate or when their partner supplements vaginal penetration with some form of clitoral stimulation.

The fact that a woman doesn't have an orgasm when she has intercourse doesn't mean that she is frigid or that there is anything wrong with her technique or her partner's technique.

ADVICE FOR WOMEN WHO HAVE DIFFICULTY REACHING ORGASM

1. Tell your partner what turns you on and off. Don't be shy. If you don't tell him he'll probably never know. At the same time encourage him to tell you what *he* likes best.

2. Try not to have sex when you are anxious or under pressure. Take the telephone off the hook if you find it difficult to ignore. Try to relax and push your problems to one side before you have sex. If you are preoccupied then your chances of having an orgasm are remote.

3. Most women find it easier to reach an orgasm if they fantasize. Try reading books with sexy scenes or watching sexy movies if you are not sure what to fantasize about. Don't be worried by your fantasies – however bizarre they may seem. There is a lot of difference between what happens in your fantasies and what actually happens in real life.

4. Be prepared to let yourself go. Many women find that dressing up for sex (for example in black stockings and suspenders) turns them on *because* it turns their partners on. You are more likely to reach orgasm if you are enjoying sex. Don't make the mistake of taking ordinary everyday sex too seriously (I am assuming that you are not having sex ONLY to have a baby).

5. If you have difficulty in reaching orgasm during sex try masturbating (see page 54). If you feel shy about using your hands, or if it doesn't seem to work, try using a vibrator (see the illustration below). Then incorporate what you have learned into your love-making.

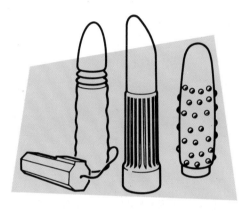

LAX VAGINA

When a woman has a baby her pelvic and vaginal muscles are put under a considerable strain – inevitably, as they have to stretch to let the baby through. It is hardly surprising that those muscles often lose some of their tone and strength.

When this happens a woman may complain that she no longer gets as much satisfaction from sex as she got before. Her partner may complain that he finds sex less satisfying too. The main problem will be that the vaginal muscles will be less able to grip the penis tightly when it enters. As a result there will be less stimulation for him and less likelihood that her labia minora will pull down on her clitoris to take her to (or at least towards) orgasm.

By deliberately exercising the muscles in and around the vagina it is possible to regain vaginal muscle tone. Follow these steps:

1. The muscles that control your vaginal walls also control the flow of urine from your bladder.

Begin your exercises by sitting on the lavatory with your legs apart and your arms resting on your thighs. Force a little urine out of your bladder. Stop almost immediately, as soon as the stream of urine has started. Use the muscles around your vagina to stop the flow. For the next few minutes continue to pass urine in short bursts, contracting your muscles to regulate or control the flow.

2. After practising like this you should be able to contract and relax the relevant muscles without needing a flow of urine to show you that you are succeeding.

3. Try exercising the same muscles while you are lying flat on your back on your bed. Undress first and make sure that the bedroom is warm and that you will not be disturbed. Put a pillow under your bottom.

4. Moisten one finger and place it gently inside your vagina. If you have any difficulty in doing this, lift up your knees and put your feet flat on the bed. While the finger is inside you, try squeezing hard with the muscles around your vagina. You should be able to feel the muscles contracting. Then let the muscles relax and go loose. If you repeat this simple exercise frequently you should be able to strengthen your vaginal muscles.

5. Without having a finger in your vagina try bearing down – as though you were trying to push a baby out of your vagina. Then, try moving the muscles the other way – so that if there was anything in the front of your vagina it would be sucked inwards. If you can find something suitable – such as a vaginal dilator – you can exercise with that.

6. Once you have tried this exercise a few times you'll know what it feels like and you will be able to exercise your muscles whatever you are doing and wherever you are. You can try it in the supermarket or on a bus, while you are doing the washing up or chatting to a friend. Before long you will have impressive vaginal muscle power, strong enough to squeeze anything that happens to be inside your vagina.

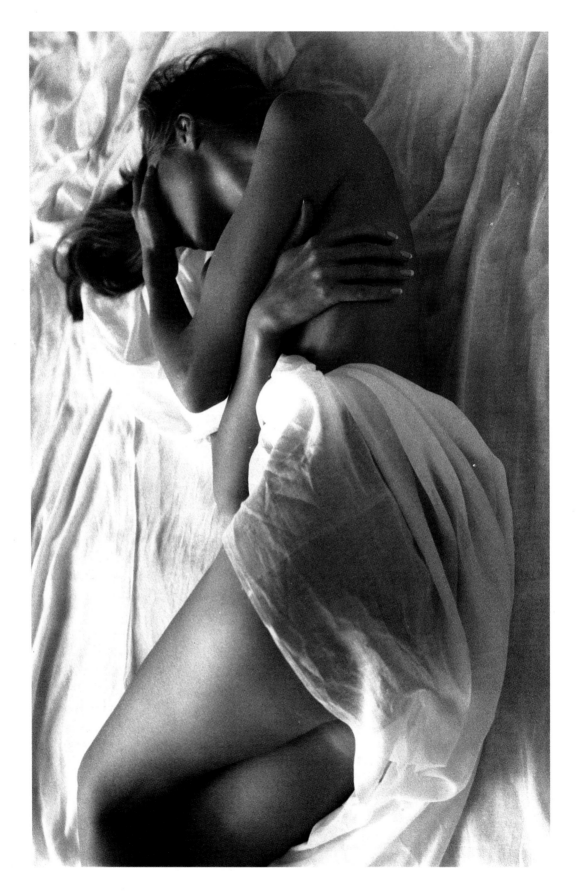

PAIN

Only a masochist enjoys sex when it hurts.

There are numerous reasons why sex may be painful: superficial pains and soreness can be caused by vaginal dryness, allergy reactions, cuts and sores or localized infections. Forgotten tampons and other objects accidentally left inside the vagina can lead to considerable discomfort. Cystitis is another possible cause of pain. A rigid hymen, an opening made too small after the repair of a tear caused by childbirth and vaginismus can also create problems.

Deeper pains may be caused by fibroids, endometriosis, chronic pelvic congestion (sometimes caused by having sex repeatedly without ever having an orgasm), ovarian cysts, a retroverted uterus, a prolapse or an infection of the cervix. If you ever find that sex is painful you should consult your doctor.

WET VAGINA

Many women complain that they produce *too much* lubrication and that when their vaginas are too moist neither they nor their partners can get proper satisfaction.

There is no medical cure for this problem. The only answer is to use a towel or strong paper tissue to wipe away the excess fluid.

BLEEDING

Any woman who notices unexplained bleeding from her vagina before, during or after sex should see her doctor for an examination.
There are several possible explanations.
• **If a virgin has had sex for the first time her hymen may have been torn, almost inevitably causing bleeding.**
• **If your partner has been rough then he may have caused some bleeding, particularly if your vagina was not properly lubricated before penetration began.**
• **In post-menopausal women, the vagina's ability to lubricate itself diminishes.**
• **Bleeding may occur if the cervix is damaged or inflamed.**

DRY VAGINA

One in five pre-menopausal women (and considerably more menopausal women) complain that their vaginas are dry and make sex uncomfortable. There are several possible causes.

Fear is one possibility (the production of lubricating substances goes down when a woman is afraid) but a lack of proper preparation is even more likely. A longer period of foreplay will usually solve the problem. If the amount of natural lubrication remains too low oils and jellies can be bought from the pharmacy. Saliva is the cheapest and most readily available lubricant.

CYSTITIS

Cystitis – an inflammation of the bladder – is extremely common among women because the female urethra (the tube that carries urine down from the bladder) is much shorter and more vulnerable to infection.

The two symptoms most commonly associated with cystitis are: a painful 'burning' sensation on passing urine and the need to pass small amounts of urine unusually frequently. Other symptoms include the passing of cloudy, discoloured or blood-stained urine.

There is a strong link between cystitis and sex, and 'honeymoon' cystitis is the name given to cystitis thought to have been caused by sex. Brides are supposed to be exceptionally vulnerable to cystitis but 'honeymoon' cystitis is certainly NOT confined to brides.

Sex can cause bladder trouble in two ways. First, if intercourse is particularly energetic the female urethra, which runs close to the vagina, may be subjected to a physical battering. Second, an infection may be passed on during sex. The problem can be minimized by:
• **experimenting with different positions**
• **making sure that both partners wash thoroughly before sex**
• **avoiding aggressive thrusting or deep penetration**
• **emptying the bladder after sex to make sure that any bacteria around the entrance to the**

urethra are washed away
• placing a pillow under the woman's buttocks during sex in the missionary position
• making sure that the vagina is well lubricated before sex

FIBROIDS

The normal, healthy uterus is made up of a huge number of powerful muscle fibres. Although no one really knows why they do it, these fibres can occasionally grow too much, forming muscle tumours known as myomata or fibroids.

Benign, and more of a nuisance than anything else, these fibroids can sometimes grow to the size of a grapefruit. Usually they are smaller, say the size of a small orange or a plum. If they are really big they can be felt from the outside and may even make a woman look pregnant.

Apart from their variation in size, fibroids fall into one or two main categories: there are those which grow into the lining of the uterus and which can therefore affect a woman's periods, and the ones which remain within the wall of the uterus. Fibroids which grow into the womb lining, which may produce some quite heavy bleeding even if they are quite small, are known as submucous or intestitial fibroids. Fibroids which remain within the uterus wall are known as sub serous. They sometimes fail to produce any symptoms at all.

One in every five women ends up growing fibroids at some time in her life. The problem is more common in women who have not had any children or who have had children late in life.

Fibroids can either be removed surgically and individually or they can be removed together with the whole uterus (hysterectomy). A myomectomy (the specific removal of a fibroid) is the most suitable operation for a young woman who may want to have children. A hysterectomy is only suitable for a woman who is certain that she will never want more children.

ENDOMETRIOSIS

Each month the cells which make up the lining of the womb (the endometrium) build up under hormonal control. If no egg is fertilized, the lining breaks down and the discharge of the cells from the womb produces a monthly bleed.

Problems can occur if the endometrial tissue is present outside the womb. If, for example, endometrial tissue is attached to the outer sides of the womb itself, is wrapped around one or both ovaries, or is fixed in the pelvis then that tissue will respond to the monthly build up of hormones in exactly the same way as the endometrial tissue inside the womb.

The cells will get thicker and thicker and finally, after expanding to their collective limit, they will then break down and bleed.

Inside the womb bleeding isn't a problem. The blood passes out through the cervix and the vagina and is discharged from the body. But when the endometrial tissue is on the other side of the womb wall problems arise. The blood cannot escape as a period bleed can. It builds up and forms cysts. And there is often a considerable amount of pain. Indeed pain is probably the most important and commonest single symptom of endometriosis. There may be pain at period time, pain during intercourse and general pain for no good reason.

Precisely why endometrial tissue develops in these wayward places is something of a mystery. But we do know that all the symptoms associated with endometriosis are very much under hormonal control. Indeed, endometriosis ceases

"Precisely why endometrial tissue develops in these wayward places is something of a mystery. But we do know that all the associated symptoms are very much under hormonal control."

to be a problem in women who have reached the menopause, and who are, therefore, undergoing hormonal changes.

Most important, perhaps, it is also known that pregnancy seems to be an effective treatment for endometriosis. It is possible to imitate the hormonal changes associated with pregnancy by giving a hormone pill.

Occasionally hormone treatment doesn't work and the endometriosis persists. When that happens the sufferer may need an operation to remove the extraneous tissue.

Endometriosis is not always easy to diagnose, but it is a fairly common problem and it should always be suspected whenever a woman develops strange pains in or around the pelvis or lower abdomen or develops pains which are worse either at period time or during intercourse.

OVARIAN CYSTS

A cyst is an enlargement or swelling that is usually filled with fluid. Ovaries commonly develop cysts which can vary from the size of a grape to the size of a melon. Most cysts are harmless but they can occasionally twist, rupture or bleed.

RETROVERTED UTERUS

Under normal circumstances the uterus is bent slightly forward, resting on the bladder and lying at an angle of ninety degrees to the vagina. Sometimes, however, the uterus is bent backwards – this is known as retroversion.

Some doctors think that a retroverted uterus can make sex painful.

PROLAPSE

Normally, the uterus sits in the abdomen with only the cervix projecting down into the upper part of the vagina. The uterus is kept in position by muscles and ligaments. Sometimes, however, the supports become weakened and the uterus falls down and into the vagina. Technically there are three stages for a prolapse.

In a first degree prolapse, the uterus falls down but stays inside the vagina.

In a second degree prolapse, the uterus stays inside the vagina for most of the time but if the sufferer coughs or sneezes it will pop outside. This can be a frightening experience as the cervix will be clearly visible.

In a third degree prolapse, the muscles which support the uterus are so weak that the uterus and the cervix remain outside all the time. When this happens the prolapsed uterus is known as a procidentia, and the main risk in this type of prolapse is that chafing will cause bleeding and a considerable amount of soreness. The vaginal walls get turned inside out too.

Since the problem is caused by a stretching and weakening of the muscles and ligaments, which normally hold the uterus in place, it is hardly surprising that prolapses are most common among women who have had a number of children. Prolapses are particularly likely to occur when labours have been long and dificult. Other factors which affect the likelihood of a prolapse are the menopause (which affects the production of natural hormones), obesity (which puts a mechanical strain on the tissues), heavy lifting (which strains and weakens the muscles), and coughing (which increases the pressure inside the abdomen and therefore helps to push the uterus out of the vagina).

There are several ways in which a prolapse can be tackled. If the muscle weakness is relatively slight then pelvic floor exercises, designed to strengthen the muscles, may help. Alternatively, a ring pessary (designed to hold the uterus in place) may be a suitable answer. Pessaries do need to be changed regularly to minimise the risk of infection. If, however, the prolapse is severe and the muscle weakness considerable, an operation will probably be needed to repair the tissues.

VAGINAL INFECTIONS

Vaginal infections can make sex painful or just uncomfortable. The two commonest causes of vaginal infection are trichomonas (see page 108) and thrush (see page 107).

CHAPTER SIX

Losing Interest In Sex

When men and women are asked to list the things that worry them most about sex they frequently put 'lack of interest' very near to the top. What many people fail to understand is that it is normal to have a decreasing interest in sex as the years go by – particularly if you share your life with one partner.

SEX AND RELATIONSHIPS

When a relationship begins sex is often extremely important. Newly weds frequently make love many times a week – often, many times a *day*. But as the weeks and months go by it is normal for that initial enthusiasm to fade. Gradually, other aspects of the relationship become increasingly important. Familiarity breeds contentment. Friendship and companionship grow in significance and, after a year or two, most married couples will privately admit that a regular sex life is less important than having someone to love, care for and share things with. Gradually, other things become more important. Work, family, hobbies and friends all start to take precedence over sex.

Unfortunately, when people are asked about how often they make love they invariably lie. People don't like admitting that they make love once a month (or even less often) and so when questioned, they say that they still make love two or three times a week.

Such white lies help to keep the myth (and the guilt) going. When the next lot of interviewees are asked how often *they* have sex they lie too. No one wants to admit that their sex life is less than 'normal'. What they do not realize is that there is a great difference between what they think is 'normal' and what really is 'normal'.

There is a story about American President Coolidge which illustrates this phenomenon extremely well.

Coolidge was visiting an American farm with his wife. Soon after their arrival the President and his wife were taken off on separate tours. When Mrs Coolidge passed the chicken pens she asked the keeper how often the rooster made love to his hens. 'Dozens of times,' answered the keeper, undoubtedly rather surprised and probably a little embarrassed. 'Please tell that to the President,' said Mrs Coolidge with a sly smile.

When Mr Coolidge's half of the tour arrived at the chicken house the keeper passed on the information. 'Same hen every time?' asked the President. 'Oh, no, Mr President!' answered the keeper. 'A different one each time.' Mr Coolidge nodded wisely. 'Please tell that to Mrs Coolidge,' he instructed the keeper.

The slowing down in the frequency of lovemaking is not peculiar to the human species. It is something that happens in other species too, and like humans it is often only the introduction of a new partner which triggers an increase in sexual activity.

At the start of any physical relationship most couples try different techniques to keep their sex life alive. But the possibilities are, in reality, limited and are often exhausted after a few months. What was once exciting becomes monotonous and other things assume greater importance. Eventually, in most relationships, a comfortable pattern develops. If the relationship is a good one – and one that will last – then sex will eventually play just a small part in keeping the

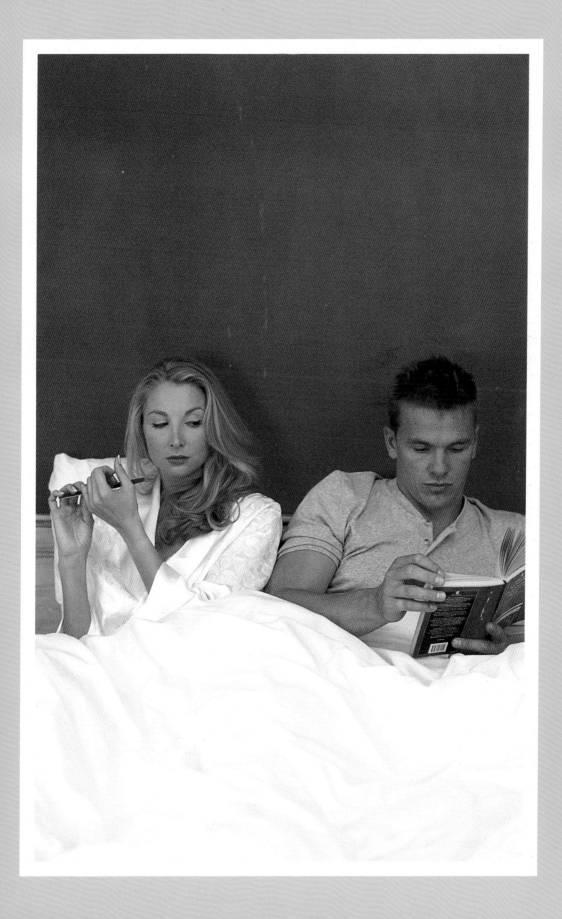

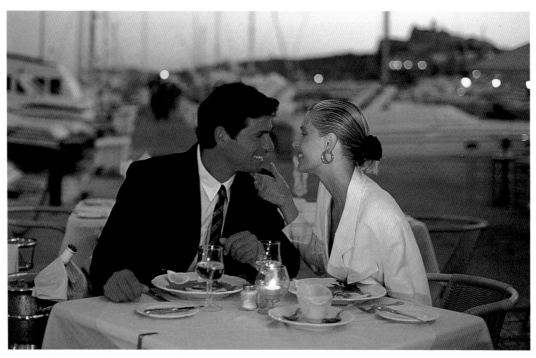

couple together. Many relationships start off based on sex but end up being based on friendship and companionship.

There is nothing at all wrong with this change. It is perfectly NORMAL.

But many people worry when they realize that they are not having sex as often as they were. They assume that there must be something wrong with the relationship. They worry that their partner does not find them attractive or does not love them. They feel inadequate. Often they look for things to blame.

If all the sparkle has gone from your relationship then you may be able to put some of it back. Flowers, candle-lit dinners, romantic weekends and lacy nightwear can put some excitement back into a well-developed relationship. But the truth is that nothing can bring back that initial sense of physical excitement that heralds the start of a sexual relationship. You will never again rediscover that feeling of insatiability and the feeling that you and your partner have invented sex.

Wise couples recognize that sexual habits and sexual patterns do change – in quality and quantity – with time. Sex may still be important and

fun but it is no longer the sole reason for living and nor is it the glue that binds the two partners together in the relationship.

Apart from a natural and inevitable lessening of interest in sex as a relationship blossoms, there are more specific (and more remediable) reasons why people lose their enthusiasm for sex.

EXHAUSTION

Stress, anxiety, tiredness and overwork are all enemies of sex. Any man or woman who is under too much pressure will, inevitably, find that his or her interest in sex will fall away rapidly. Tiredness and exhaustion mean that going to bed becomes a chance to rest or to sleep, rather than an opportunity to experiment with new sexual positions!

This problem affects millions of men and women whose daily commitments are so great that sex is gradually pushed to one side. The more determined, the more ambitious and the more hard-working an individual is, the greater the chance that his or her sex life will be pushed to one side.

If your sex life has been crushed by your other interests, and it worries you, then you can

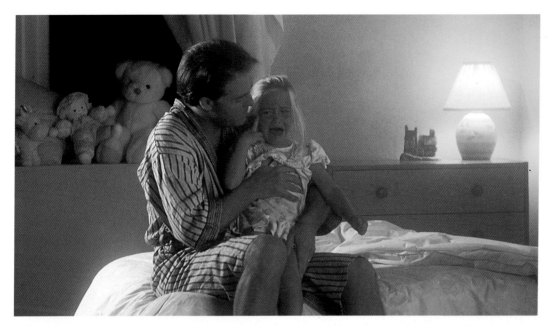

do something about it. The best way to deal with the problem is to sort out your priorities and to allocate your time more carefully.

DEPRESSION

Sex drive is linked closely to mood and a sudden or gradual loss of interest in sex may be associated with a feeling of depression.

There may be psychological causes for the depression (worry about specific problems such as work, children or money) or the depression may be caused by a physical problem (for example, the sort of hormonal changes that can take place during or after childbirth or the menopause). When there is a cause for a mood change then the solution is, of course, to deal

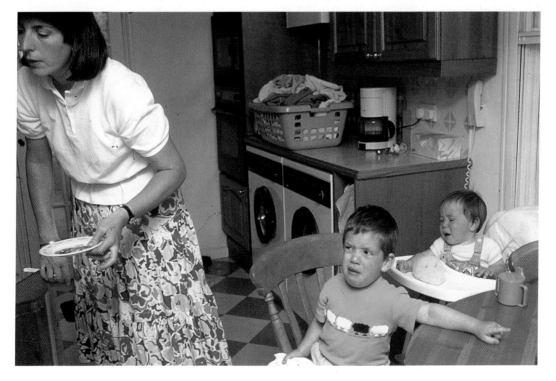

with that underlying cause. Only then will interest in sex be restored. If you feel depressed for any reason then you should visit your doctor and ask for help, advice and treatment.

DRUG THERAPY

If your interest in sex has disappeared or been reduced AND you are taking a drug prescribed by your doctor or a drug that you have bought from the pharmacy, then the chances are high that the drug is responsible for the changes in your sex life.

It is impossible to provide a full and up-to-date list of the drugs that can affect sexual interest and ability (the list changes constantly) but some of the types of drug commonly associated with this problem include:

- **tranquillizers**
- **sleeping tablets**
- **drugs for anxiety**
- **anti-depressants**
- **drugs used to control blood pressure**
- **drugs used to treat heart disease**
- **drugs used to treat headaches**
- **drugs used to treat fluid retention**

This list is not by any means comprehensive.

If you think that your sex life could have been affected by drugs that have been prescribed by your doctor or that you have bought from a pharmacy, then you should consult your doctor or pharmacist straight away.

Do NOT stop the suspected drug until you have spoken to your doctor or pharmacist because this may cause additional problems. If

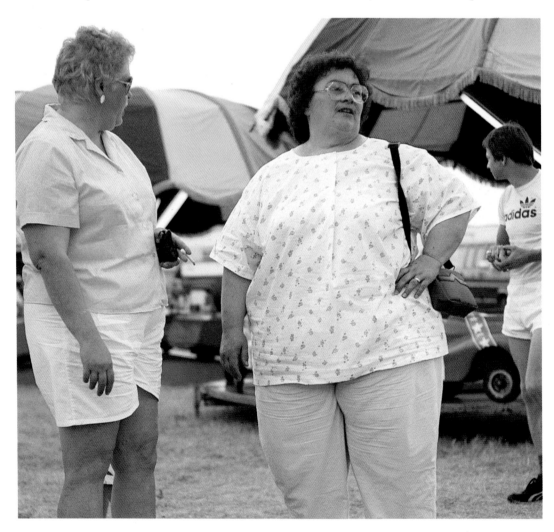

you need to stop taking the drug you may need to do so slowly. But if the drug you are taking could be responsible, there may be an alternative that you can try that does not produce this unfortunate side effect.

CELIBACY

If you haven't had sex for several months then your natural sexual urges will gradually become weaker and weaker. People who are celibate (either through choice, because they are separated from their partner, or because they cannot find a suitable partner) often find that as time goes by their interest in sex falls.

There is a simple physical explanation for what may seem to be an alarming phenomenon. If you haven't had sex for a while then the quantity of sex hormones circulating in your body will have fallen. Eventually the level will become so low that your interest in and enthusiasm for sex will also fall. However, once you start having sex again your circulating sex hormone levels will rise – and then you'll gradually recover your interest in sex.

REPULSION

It may sound cruel to mention this, but it's a fact of life and to ignore it would be pointless. As we get older and more secure and settled in a relationship we tend to take things for granted. We often let ourselves go.

When we are young we make a real effort to look at our best. We buy fashionable clothes and we dress carefully. We look after our hair and our skin and we try to control our weight. But as the years go by these things seem to become less and less important.

He may become fat, bald and scruffy. He may not bother to shave at the weekends.

She may become comfortably 'plump'; always dressing in sensible clothes and making no effort with her hair or her make-up unless she is going out to meet friends.

You may not think that these things matter. And in some relationships they do not. True

love is often blind. But if a relationship is rocky or under pressure, appearances can be extremely important to both partners.

FEAR OF DISCOVERY

If you have no place where you can make love in comfort and private then your ability to enjoy sex will be severely affected by your fear of discovery. It is difficult to relax (an essential prerequisite to a successful orgasm) if you are worried about someone opening the living room door or shining a torch in through your car window. In such circumstances, it is not unusual for sexual interest to decline altogether.

FEAR OF PREGNANCY

Neither partner will be able to relax or to enjoy a proper sexual relationship if either one is worried about an unwanted pregnancy. There is advice about contraception on pages 96–101.

FEAR OF DISEASE

Similarly, neither partner will be able to relax if either one is worried about contracting a sexually transmitted disease. There is information on (and advice about avoiding) sexually transmitted diseases on pages 102–109.

FEAR OF INADEQUACY

Thousands of perfectly sensible, perfectly good-looking and otherwise sane and confident individuals suffer agonies because of fears that their bodies or their sexual skills are inadequate.

The first part of the problem is undoubtedly inspired by the photographs of abnormally physically endowed women (and occasionally men) in magazines and tabloid newspapers. Female models who pose professionally for the camera are usually either boyishly thin (if they are being hired to sell dresses) or absurdly and abnormally voluptuous (if they being hired to grace the pages of mens' magazines). It is not surprising that looking at these photographs gives many women an inferiority complex.

The second part of the problem is inspired

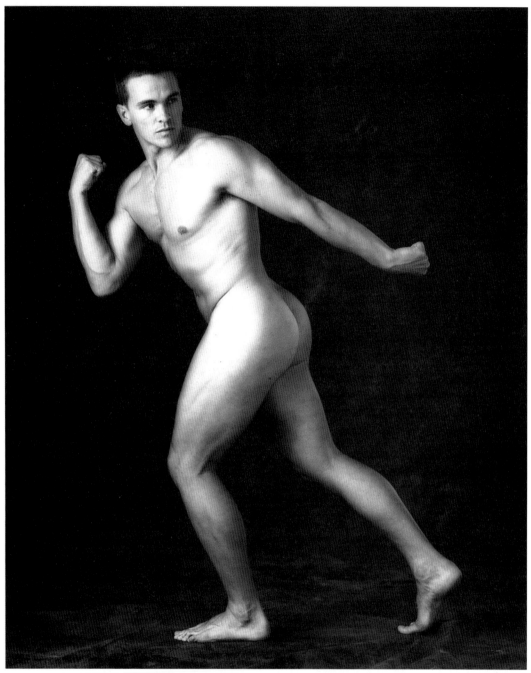

Advertising, the media, and the fashion world have led people to believe that perfection is normal

partly by those commentators and journalists who write so glibly and easily about the (imaginary) sex lives of the rich and famous; partly by the 'experts' who, when they write about sexual matters usually do so with a startling confidence and an unerring ability to raise expectations, offering their readers hopes and aspirations that are incompatible with reality; and partly by novelists who write about sex in a way that is quite divorced from reality. Women who fail to achieve multiple orgasms every time they have sex are encouraged to believe that there must be something wrong either with them or with their partners, and men who cannot sustain an erec-

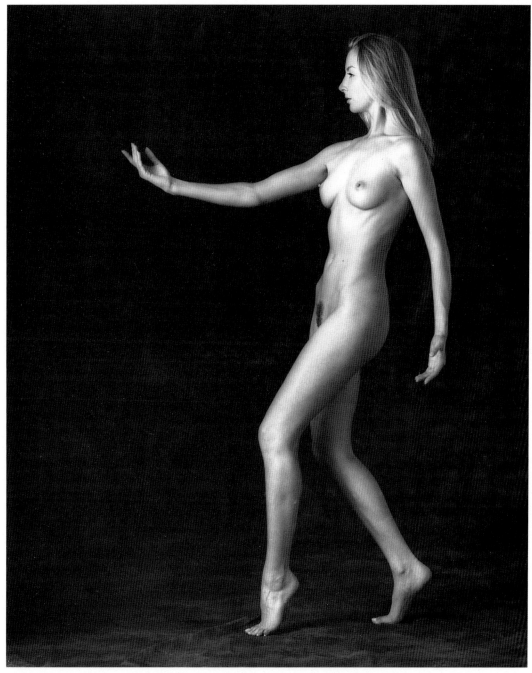

Women are expected to be models of perfection, either boyishly thin or sexily voluptuous

tion for long enough for their partners to achieve orgasm are led to believe (quite incorrectly) that they are sexually incompetent.

The wit and the romance and the fun have, to a large extent, been removed from sex and replaced by standards, rights and expectations. We may be more enlightened and less prudish than our ancestors but we have created our own range of social and sexual stresses. Guilt, self-doubt and inadequacy produce either frigidity or impotence or a total disinterest and disinclination to take any interest in sex. No one points out that sex is just one small part of an understanding and enjoyable relationship.

CHAPTER SEVEN

How To Get Pregnant

Infertility is the medical problem that most commonly takes young adults to the doctor. At least one in ten couples don't seem to be able to start the baby they both badly want. Sometimes expert help may be needed at an infertility clinic. But not always.

WHEN EVERYTHING GOES RIGHT

Each month changing hormone levels trigger the release of an egg from the thousands stored in a healthy woman's two ovaries. The release of an egg is known as ovulation and this normally takes place in between two menstrual periods. Once an egg has been released it travels down one of the Fallopian tubes.

When a healthy male partner ejaculates, millions of tadpole-shaped sperm are fired into the vagina at tremendous speed. Each individual sperm carries half a blueprint for a baby. The other half of the blueprint is stored in the woman's egg.

However, although it takes only one sperm to do the job, sperm may come in teams of around 200,000,000. Some of the 199,999,999 unlucky sperm are designed not to rush for the egg but to help the chosen one get to the right position on time. When one sperm is close to the egg, some of the remainder will, for example, link together to form a barrier stopping more sperm rushing on and getting in the way.

Most of the sperm die in the vagina, but after a struggle for a couple of hours a few million manage to get through the cervix and into the womb. Once inside they swim on for another five or six hours. At the upper end of the womb the sperm have a choice of two tubes. If they swim along one they will find an egg which one of them may fertilize. If they swim along the other they will experience a lingering death.

Inside the Fallopian tube, the sperm have to swim against a current which will eventually help force the fertilized egg on its journey down the tube into the womb. When the successful sperm finally struggles inside the waiting egg, the remainder will die.

THINGS THAT CAN GO WRONG

There are many possible causes of infertility, for there are many things that can go wrong in this complicated scenario.

Among women, the most frequent problems are a failure of ovulation and a blockage of the Fallopian tubes. Among men, the most common problems are a failure to produce sperm of good enough quality or a failure to produce sperm in sufficient numbers. Infertility is often a symptom or a consequence of some other disorder. For example, general disorders such as diabetes or thyroid problems can cause infertility; sexually transmitted diseases can result in later infertility and, very occasionally, a woman may develop anti-sperm antibodies.

When a man doesn't produce enough sperm or produces sperm of inferior quality, the basic cause may be an old infection or an accident. Mumps is a common cause of male sterility. When a woman fails to ovulate, the cause may be general (such as a loss of weight) or specific (such as endometriosis, see pages 78–79).

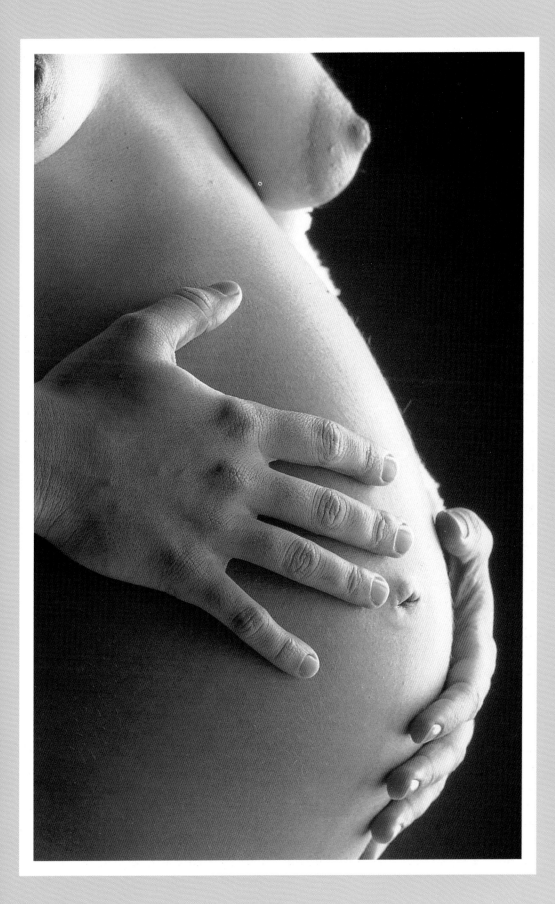

Sometimes infertility may result from the fact that sperm haven't had a fair chance of meeting an egg. The couple who make love once a year are less likely to start a family quickly than the couple who make love every day of the month. If he is impotent or ejaculates prematurely then she isn't likely to get pregnant either.

Finally, there are still an astonishing number of men and women who have no idea how babies are made. I have met couples who thought that babies were made by depositing sperm in the woman's navel (one woman thought that putting sticking plaster over her navel would act as a contraceptive). I know a woman who made her husband take the contraceptive pill because they both enjoyed oral sex (she pointed out that it is called the oral contraceptive) and couples whose knowledge and understanding of conception is a tribute to centuries of repression.

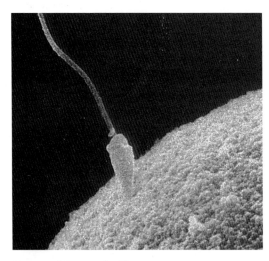

A successful sperm fertilizes an egg

THE TEN MOST LIKELY CAUSES OF INFERTITLITY

1. She is not ovulating properly.
2. He is not producing enough sperm – or his sperm are abnormal.
3. She has Fallopian tubes that have been damaged by infection.
4. He has undescended testicles.
5. He has testicles damaged by injury or infection and do not produce sperm properly.
6. She has endometriosis.
7. He is impotent or ejaculates prematurely.
8. They do not have sex at the right times.
9. They do not have sex often enough.
10. She has produced antibodies to his sperm.

WHOSE PROBLEM HIS OR HERS?

The woman is usually blamed when a couple cannot start a family. But it is just as likely to be his fault as hers.

If 10 couples can't have children:
• **In 3 cases it will be HIS fault**
• **In 3 cases it will be HER fault.**
• **In 2 cases it will be BOTH their faults.**
• **In 2 cases the reason will be a mystery.**

HOW LIKELY ARE YOU TO GET PREGNANT? (FOR WOMEN ONLY)

Answer Yes or No to all these questions.
1. Do you have a good idea of when you ovulate?
2. Do you make a real effort to make love at or around the time of ovulation?
3. Are your periods reasonably regular?
4. Have you taken the contraceptive pill at any time in the last three months?
5. Do you avoid sex at times when you know that you cannot possibly get pregnant in order to preserve your partner's sperm for when you might get pregnant?
6. Do you suffer from any medical illness which you think might affect your chances of becoming pregnant? (General disorders such as thyroid disease and diabetes or specific gynaecological problems, such as endometriosis or ovarian cysts, can all have an affect on fertility.)
7. Does your partner have any medical problems such as undescended testicles or swellings in or around his testicles, which might affect your chances of getting pregnant?
8. Are you currently trying to lose weight?
9. Have you recently taken up any kind of strenuous exercise programme?

10. Are you currently breast-feeding?

11. Are you under eighteen or over forty years of age?

12. Do you feel under a great deal of stress or pressure?

13. Do you usually stay in bed – lying down – after having sex?

14. Does your partner wear tight-fitting underwear and/or trousers?

15. Have you ever been pregnant before or has your partner ever made another woman pregnant?

Now check your score:

Score 1 point for answering YES to the following questions:

1, 2, 3, 5, 13, 15

Score 1 point for answering NO to the following questions:

4, 6, 7, 8, 9, 10, 11, 12, 14

> **If you scored 15, then you are doing everything you can to get pregnant.**
> **If you scored between 12 and 14, be careful if you don't want to get pregnant.**
> **If you scored between 6 and 11, then there are several things you could do to increase your chances of having a baby.**
> **If you scored 5 or less, then you may need help to get pregnant. Read this chapter carefully to find out what you should do – and why – to increase your chances of becoming pregnant.**

HOW TO BEAT INFERTILITY

Here are some practical pieces of advice that should prove helpful:

1. A woman will only get pregnant if his sperm and her egg are both in the right place at the right time. Remember that:

• **The first day of a menstrual cycle begins on the first day that a menstrual bleed starts. A cycle ends on the day before the next bleed starts. Ovulation usually (but not always)** occurs twelve to sixteen days before the beginning of a menstrual bleed.

• **An egg can usually be fertilized between twelve and twenty-four hours after ovulation.**

• **His sperm can (in theory at least) fertilize eggs up to five days after ejaculation, as long as her cervical mucus remains wet, sticky and in a 'fertile' condition. In practice, sperm usually have a shorter active life than this.**

2. Sperm are very susceptible to heat. To ensure that his sperm are kept in the best possible condition, he should avoid wearing tight jeans or tight underpants, should keep out of very hot baths and saunas and should sit with his legs wide apart as often as possible.

3.. After sex she should stay in bed for half an hour, draw up her knees and put a pillow under her bottom. All these things help increase the chance of sperm getting into and through the cervix. The more sperm that get into the womb the greater the chance of a pregnancy ensuing.

4. A change in a woman's exercise pattern can reduce her chances of getting pregnant. A woman who takes up jogging or aerobics may not ovulate regularly.

5.. Stress and worry can result in a failure to ovulate and, therefore, a reduction in the chances of getting pregnant. There is considerable evidence to show that a woman's ability to conceive depends upon her state of mind. Hormonal changes are easily influenced by all sorts of psychological factors. For example, if a woman is worried about something her period may be late. If a woman suspects that fears or doubts are the cause of infertility, then she should try to learn how to relax, build up her self-confidence and replace anxieties with firm hopes and plans for the future.

6. If a woman's weight changes substantially, either up or down, then that can reduce her chances of getting pregnant.

7. Some experts claim that it is possible for a woman to decide when she is most likely to become pregnant by studying the consistency of her own cervical mucus. The type of mucus produced by the small glands in the cervix changes throughout the menstrual cycle. Immediately after the end of a menstrual bleed, the amount of cervical mucus produced will probably be quite low, with the result that the area around and just inside the vagina will feel dry and may be sore during sex or when a tampon is used. (By absorbing all moisture the tampon may exacerbate this dryness.) Then a very sticky type of mucus will be produced. This mucus, which does not contain much moisture, tends to leave a light yellow stain on white underwear. Finally, closer to ovulation the cervical mucus will be creamier and whiter. As ovulation approaches, the mucus will become wetter and clearer. The amount produced will increase too. The mucus, which at this time of the cycle has the appearance and texture of raw egg white, can be stretched out between the fingers. Most woman ovulate at the time of the month when their mucus is at its wettest.

7. A woman's basal body temperature (the temperature of her body at rest) changes as her hormone levels change during her monthly cycle. At the end of a menstrual period the body temperature (taken first thing in the morning, preferably while you are still lying in bed) will usually be somewhere in the range 96°F to 97.4°F. After ovulation has taken place, the basal

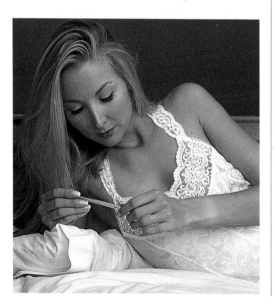

body temperature will rise slightly by between 0.3° F and 1.0°F. When the basal body temperature has remained at this higher level for three days, you know that an egg has been released from one of your ovaries.

9. At, or around the time, when they ovulate some women notice symptoms which are similar to the symptoms normally associated with the pre-menstrual syndrome. These symptoms normally last for just a day or two and the commonest include:
- **slight irritability**
- **an unusually clear complexion, with a reduction in the amount of oil in the skin**
- **some fluid retention, leading to a bloated feeling and slight breast tenderness**

10. Some women notice a pain or an ache in their pelvic region at or around the time of ovulation. Others notice a small amount of bleeding or 'spotting' at ovulation. Often all that women actually notice is a tiny spot of blood marking their underwear.

11. Many women notice that their interest in and enthusiasm for sex changes slightly during ovulation. Some feel more interested in sex – others less interested.

12. Some women feel more energetic just before or at ovulation. Women also sometimes claim that their senses of smell, taste and vision are sharper during ovulation.

QUESTIONS ABOUT FERTILITY

How old are you and your partner?
If you are over 40 then your chances of getting pregnant are dramatically reduced. Only half of all women over the age of 40 are still fertile and pregnancy is rare over the age of 45. Age affects men less but it is a factor – the older he is the more likely there are to be problems.

How long have you been trying to conceive?
If you have been trying for less than six months then there is still an excellent chance that you will get pregnant without any help. It is often

more difficult to get pregnant than you might think, and it can take time. Your egg and his sperm have to be in the right place together at the right time. If you have been trying to have a baby for more than two years without any success, then you should talk to your doctor now. If you have been trying to get pregnant for between six months and two years and you are in your late twenties or older, then you should also talk to your doctor now. If you are still in your early or mid twenties, you can wait until you've been trying for two years (unless you're desperate to get pregnant now).

Has your partner ever made another woman pregnant?

If he has, then the chances are that he is fertile and you are not. Or there could be some problem about the timing of your love-making.

Have you ever had a baby or been made pregnant by another partner?

If the answer is YES, then the chances are that you are fertile and your partner is not. Or there could be some problem about the timing of your love-making.

How often do you make love?

As long as you make love once a month, WHEN you make love is much more important than how often you make love.

Are you absolutely certain that you know HOW to make a baby?

You'd be surprised how many apparently sensible men and women aren't entirely sure what goes where and does what. If you have any doubts at all read the introductory chapter to this book again and maybe talk to your doctor.

Does your partner suffer from impotence or premature ejaculation?

If he does then you must deal with this problem first. Talk to him. Talk to your doctor. Both these common male problems are usually 'men-tal' rather than 'physical'. Anxiety and stress can cause them both. See pages 62–69 for advice.

Do you find sex painful or difficult?

You must deal with the cause if you do. Dryness is one of the most common causes of pain during sex (use a lubricant such as saliva). See page 70–79 for other causes of pain during sex.

Have either of you ever had a sexually transmitted infection?

Sexually transmitted infections can affect the sexual or reproductive organs. Gonorrhoea, tuberculosis and salpingitis (inflammation of a Fallopian tube) could affect your ability to conceive. Gonorrhoea, non-specific urethritis or mumps could affect HIS ability to father a baby.

Has he got – and has he always had – two normal-sized testes?

If one or both of his testicles is (are) undescended or if he has (or has had) any swelling or lump in his scrotum, then his ability to make you pregnant may be affected. His doctor should be able to tell you both what the chances are.

Have you ever had a termination of a previous pregnancy or an ectopic pregnancy?

It is possible that your body could have been affected (for example your Fallopian tubes could be blocked). Talk to your doctor.

Have you ever had surgery on an ovary or have you ever had a complicated case of appendicitis?

Talk to your doctor about whether or not your surgery or your illness could have contributed to infertility.

When do you make love?

Are there any regular times each month when you never have sex? Maybe because one of you is always away on business? Maybe there are religious reasons? Or maybe you always have visitors at certain times each month. If you are going to get pregnant, then you must make love when you are likely to be ovulating rather than when you fancy sex or when it is convenient.

SPECIAL PROBLEMS WHICH CAN AFFECT YOUR CHANCES OF PREGNANCY

1. Losing weight can stop you ovulating – particularly if you lose weight rapidly.

2. If you gain weight – particularly over a short space of time – that can reduce your chances of getting pregnant too.

3. Illness – even a cold – can affect whether you ovulate or not.

4. If you have been taking the contraceptive pill, then you will probably not get pregnant straight after you stop. Ovulation may not take place until some weeks or even months after you stop taking the pill. The length of time you must wait will depend on the type of pill you were taking, the length of time you were taking it for and your body.

5. If you are breast-feeding, it is less likely that you will get pregnant.

6. If you are in your late 30s or your 40s then you may not ovulate every month as you approach the menopause. When a woman goes for twelve months without menstruating, then her chances of getting pregnant are very low.

7. A change in exercise patterns can reduce your chances of getting pregnant. If you take up a new exercise you may not ovulate regularly. Normally your body will adapt to a new exercise pattern in a few months, but if you have taken up an unusually heavy exercise routine your chances of getting pregnant may be affected.

8. Travel, particularly for long distances, may reduce your chances of getting pregnant.

9. Stress, worry and anxiety can result in a failure of ovulation and a reduction in your chances of getting pregnant.

10. Occasionally, instead of an egg being released from an ovary a cyst develops. If you have an ovarian cyst your chances of ovulating normally and getting pregnant may be reduced.

YOUR MIND CAN HELP YOU GET PREGNANT

A woman's ability to conceive may depend upon her state of mind.

In some primitive tribes, women do not conceive until they are married and it is socially acceptable for them to have babies. This 'rule' of nature applies however many sexual partners a woman has and however long she may have sex without any form of contraceptive.

Startling though this may be, evidence from developed countries suggests that it isn't as far fetched as it appears. There are many women who claim that they conceived very quickly after deciding that the time was right for them to have children. Hormonal changes are easily influenced by psychological factors and conception can be controlled by your state of mind.

To take full advantage of the power of your mind:

1. Try to learn how to relax both your body and your mind. The better you can deal with stress, the more you are likely to ovulate normally and to conceive quickly. My book on stress (in this series) contains all the information you are likely to need.

2. Fear can make you infertile, so try to eradicate your fears about pregnancy by learning as much as you can about all the changes that take place during pregnancy.

3. Build up your self-confidence and think positively. Try to think of the ways in which a pregnancy will enhance your life, your relationship and your appearance.

4. 'Negative' thoughts can stop you getting pregnant. Try to decide if you could be harbouring any doubts or fears which might impair your body's willingness to get pregnant. Are you certain that your partner wants to have a baby? Are you worried that having a baby might affect your career or your figure? If you can think of any possible problem which might be worrying you – even subconsciously – try to deal with your anxieties as directly and as honestly as you can. Talk about the future to your partner and your friends. Make up your mind positively and try to replace all doubts and anxieties with firm hopes and plans for the future.

THE EXPERTS

If you have real difficulty in getting pregnant then your doctor will probably refer you to a specialist infertility clinic.

At the clinic the doctors will probably:
• Take a full medical and personal history from you and your partner.
• Perform a general physical examination on you both.
• Do blood tests to check your hormones and general health.
• Take a sample of the mucus from your cervix (probably a few hours after you and your partner have had sex).
• Examine a sample of your partner's sperm.
• Perform a laparoscopy (a thin, bendable telescope will be pushed into your abdomen through a tiny incision).

The treatment recommended will, of course, depend upon the results. Several different types of treatment are available.
• Drugs such as clomiphene, given by mouth, will increase a woman's chances of producing an egg ready for fertilization. The only snag is that the drug sometimes works too well and there is a risk that a would-be mother will find herself having six or even more.

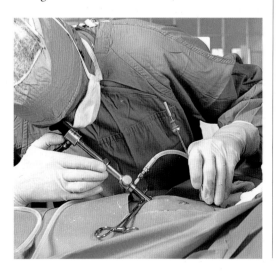

• If a Fallopian tube is damaged then surgery may be needed to repair the damage. Approximately one-fifth of all infertile women have blocked Fallopian tubes. Modern microsurgical techniques enable doctors to unblock the tubes in fifty per cent of women. Alternatively, new Fallopian tubes can sometimes be transplanted into the woman's body.
• If your partner is impotent or his sperm count is low then doctors may prepare a special sample and put this directly into your womb. This is called artificial insemination. A small syringe is used to inject the sperm into your womb. If this technique is repeated every month at ovulation, between sixty per cent and seventy-five per cent of women will get pregnant.
• If your partner's sperm seem too weak (or there aren't enough of them), then you may be offered the opportunity of using sperm provided by an anonymous donor. Some centres try to match the height and hair colour of the donor to the height and hair colour of the male partner.
• In some countries women will 'lease' out their bodies and allow themselves to be made pregnant by the would-be father. If the would-be mother has her own eggs (but has other problems) then one of her eggs may be implanted into the surrogate mother's womb. The theory is that at the end of the pregnancy, the surrogate woman will hand over the baby in return for a cheque. However, there are many legal, moral and emotional problems associated with this technique.
• If a Fallopian tube blockage cannot be overcome, an egg may be taken out of the woman's body and fertilized by her partner's sperm in the laboratory. This is what is known as a 'test-tube baby'. Your egg and your partner's sperm will be brought together for fertilization in the laboratory and then implanted into your womb to develop, so you can give birth to the baby in the normal way.
• Men who cannot father babies can sometimes be helped with male hormones which increase the number of sperm they make.

CHAPTER EIGHT

How Not To Get Pregnant

Modern contraceptive techniques are safer and more effective than those of the past. But it is still vital that couples who don't want a family know what is available.

ANCIENT CONTRACEPTIVES

Egyptian women were mixing honey and crocodile dung into contraceptive pessaries four thousand years ago. Arabian women made contraceptives from pomegranate pulps treated with alum and rocksalt, and the Greek author Aristotle described a concoction, consisting of cedar oil, frankincense and olive oil. During the sixteenth century Japanese men wore sheaths made of tortoiseshell, horn or leather. European men wore sheaths made of moistened linen. Chinese women used to cover the entrances to their wombs with discs of oiled tissue paper. In Persia women who didn't want to get pregnant were advised to take nine backward jumps after sex. Coitus interruptus – in which the male partner withdraws just before he ejaculates – was widely practised by the Hebrews and is probably the oldest known form of birth control.

Below are some of the best-known contraceptives available today.

NATURAL FAMILY PLANNING

If fertilization is to take place, the sperm and the egg must be in roughly the same place at roughly the same time. Since the egg is released at ovulation, which normally takes place roughly midway between menstrual bleeds, it is possible to estimate when conception is most likely to take place. And by the same reckoning it is possible to estimate when conception is least likely to take place.

An egg can live for about two days and sperm have a practical lifespan of a similar length. Theoretically, this means that if sperm can be kept out of the vagina for two days each side of ovulation, then it is very unlikely that a pregnancy will occur.

Ovulation normally happens between twelve and sixteen days before the beginning of a menstrual bleed. So those who favour natural family planning (also known as the rhythm method) suggest that sex be avoided between the tenth and the twentieth days of the cycle – as long as the cycle is regular.

Some experts claim that you can tell when ovulation takes place by measuring body temperature. The body temperature of a woman goes down slightly and then up slightly when an egg is released, so daily temperature readings will, in theory at least, help identify the point of ovulation. Another technique depends on the fact that the mucus in the vagina becomes wetter and more transparent at ovulation (see page 92).

THE CONTRACEPTIVE PILL

The combined contraceptive pill is probably the most effective contraceptive there is (with the exception, of course, of sterilisation). It contains a mixture of oestrogen and progestogen (the two basic female hormones) and works in three ways.

First, it stops the ovaries producing their own hormones and therefore stops ovulation – and the release of eggs.

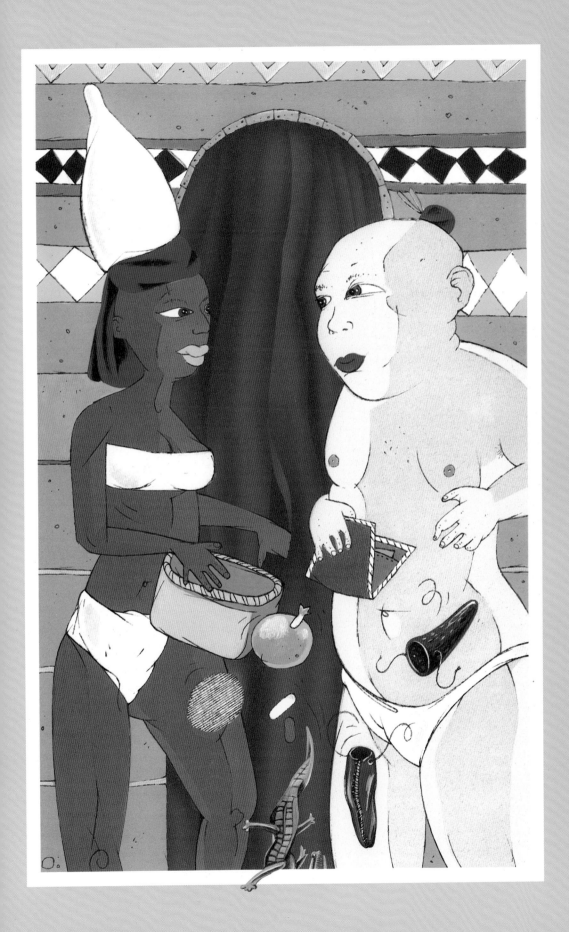

THE MENSTRUAL CYCLE

EXAMPLE: 28 DAY CYCLE | OVULATION

| 1 | 2 | 3 | 4 | 5 | 6 | 7 | 8 | 9 | 10 | 11 | 12 | 13 | 14 | 15 | 16 | 17 | 18 | 19 | 20 | 21 | 22 | 23 | 24 | 25 | 26 | 27 | 28 | 1 | 2 | 3 | 4 | 5 | 6 | 7 |

FIRST DAY OF PERIOD   THE FERTILE TIME

Second, it also changes the lining of the womb or uterus, so that if an egg does manage to escape and get fertilized it won't stand much of a chance of getting properly embedded.

Finally, the contraceptive pill also thickens the cervical mucus and makes it more difficult for sperm to get into the uterus.

There are three types of contraceptive pill.

The combined pill: contains a mixture of oestrogen and progestogen and is by far the most widely prescribed of all contraceptive pills. In recent years, low dose combined pills have been introduced which are much safer but just as effective as the older pills. If you have been taking a pill for years without having it changed, it would be worth checking with your doctor to see if there is a lower dose pill you could take. Most doctors now agree that there are some risks with the contraceptive pill – and the higher dose pills are the most likely to cause problems. Women most at risk are over thirty-five years old, smoke and have a personal or family history of heart disease.

It is the two hormones working together in the combined pill which produce the side effects and, since the proportions of oestrogen and progestogen in different pills vary, so do the side effects. The most common effects produced by the combined contraceptive pill include: acne, weight gain, headaches, sore and swollen breasts, swollen legs, vaginal discharge, nausea, depression and bleeding between periods.

In a very small number of women the contraceptive pill can cause severe illness. You should stop your pill and see your doctor straight away if you notice any of these symptoms: severe pain or swelling in your calf, bad chest pains, stomach pains, breathlessness, fainting, fits, speech defects, an inability to see clearly, bleeding after intercourse or any other unexplained bleeding, any sudden numbing or weakness, jaundice, any generalized skin rash or headaches. Most of these symptoms will be harmless but do see your doctor anyway. Any woman taking the pill should see her doctor at least once, preferably twice a year for a check-up, which should include a blood pressure check. You can help yourself by learning to examine your own breasts and by reporting any unusual bleeding, pain, discharge or other symptoms to your doctor straight away. Remember that contraceptive pills do not always mix well with other pills. Some antibiotics, tranquillizers and pain killers can counteract the effects of the pill. Check with your doctor if you need to take any drugs while you are on the pill. If you want to get pregnant then I suggest that you stop your pill six months in advance to give your own hormones a chance to get back to normal. And do not breast-feed while taking the pill since the hormones could get through to your breast milk. Do remember that when you stop taking a contraceptive pill your periods may be erratic for a month or two.

The progestogen-only pill: slightly safer than the combined pill but not as effective. It is usually taken without a break and must be taken at the same time each day. Because it contains no oestrogen, it is safer than the combined pill for older women and for women who smoke.

The triphasic pill: contains variable doses of oestrogen and progestogen and is said to have fewer side effects than the combined pill. It seems safe and effective.

Whichever contraceptive pill you decide to take, you should make sure that you read the instructions carefully and you should ask your doctor for advice and help if you have any doubts or queries.

SPERMICIDAL CREAMS

Chemicals which kill sperm can be bought as creams, pessaries, tablets, foams and aerosols. They are messy and of doubtful effectiveness, although some doctors recommend their use with condoms and they should be used with diaphragms. Used by themselves, however, spermicidal substances are probably too much of a gamble to be regarded as an effective or reliable means of contraception.

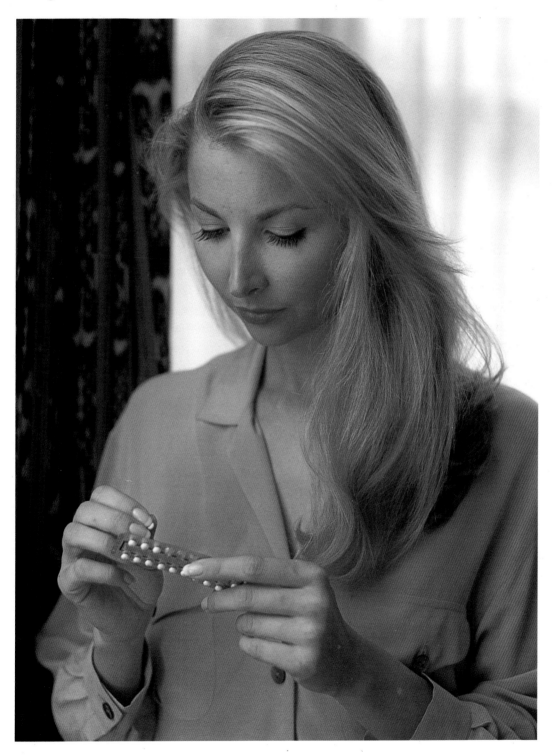

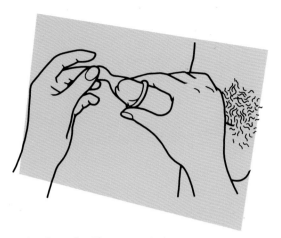

Condoms should put onto the erect penis

CONDOMS

Also known as the sheath, the condom is the only mass market contraceptive designed for use by men. The main disadvantage is that since it means pulling a thin layer of rubber over the penis it reduces sensation for both partners. However, the condom is probably the most widely used contraceptive in the world today, with over 100,000,000 people using them regularly. Condoms are useful for unplanned moments; they are convenient; they can be bought by either sex; they are readily available in most parts of the world; they produce very few side effects, they can help to delay orgasm if he suffers from premature ejaculation; they are cheap; and they provide good protection against sexually transmitted diseases.

A condom will only work properly if used properly. It should be put onto the penis as soon as the penis becomes erect (some couples make this part of their foreplay; she 'dresses' his penis as soon as possible) and removed after ejaculation and before the penis goes limp again. Artificial lubricants should not be used since they may weaken the material. If she has particularly powerful vaginal muscles she should be careful (particularly in the woman on top positions) since she may succeed in sucking the condom off his penis. When the condom fails to provide protection it is usually because of over-eagerness or carelessness.

Wearing a condom makes good sense. In addition to providing some protection against the transmission of HIV and other sexually transmitted diseases, a condom provides protection against an unwanted pregnancy.

CERVICAL CAP

Caps come in several different shapes. They can look like a large thimble or a domed hat and fit over the cervix to prevent sperm passing out of the vagina and into the womb. Because the cap was invented by a doctor from Holland, it is also commonly known as a dutch cap. The major advantage of the cervical cap over the condom is that it doesn't interfere with anyone's pleasure. The main disadvantage is that it doesn't provide much protection against infection. If put in during a menstrual period it will temporarily halt the flow of blood. Custom-made cervical caps are now available which contain a one-way valve and which can be left in position for months at a time. The valve allows menstrual fluid to flow out but doesn't allow sperm to pass through.

DIAPHRAGM

The diaphragm is a soft rubber disc fitted with a metal spring. Like the cap the diaphragm acts as a physical barrier, stopping the sperm from getting into the womb. It needs to be put into position before sex and left there until afterwards. A spermicide should always be used with a diaphragm.

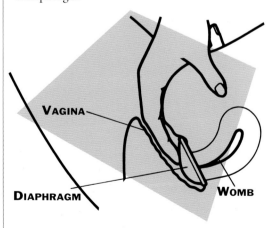

VAGINA

DIAPHRAGM

WOMB

The diaphragm should be inserted before sex

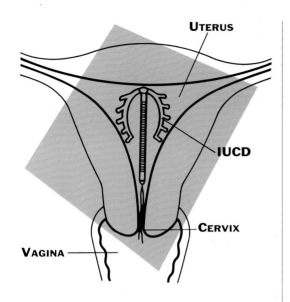

UTERUS

IUCD

CERVIX

VAGINA

INTRA-UTERINE CONTRACEPTIVE DEVICE (IUCD)

The IUCD consists of a small piece of curved plastic or metal which is put into the womb to stop a baby developing. Many women find them to be safe, effective, comfortable and convenient. They can be left in place for a year and are not usually displaced by tampons, bleeding or sex. They do not interfere with sexual pleasure and it is fairly easy to check that they are still in place by feeling for the thread which should poke out through the cervix. Occasionally, the IUCD can cause heavy bleeding, a vaginal discharge and cramp-like pains, and very rarely an IUCD may work its way through the wall of the womb and into the abdomen. You must see your doctor if you want to have an IUCD inserted.

COITUS INTERRUPTUS

The theory is that if he takes his penis out of her vagina before he ejaculates then she won't get pregnant. This very old-fashioned method costs nothing and is widely used but *isn't* very efficient. Just before ejaculation a few drops of liquid usually leak out from the end of the penis, and these drops may contain some sperm. Many pregnancies among women over the age of forty result from the use of this method. This happens because she is too old to take the pill and too embarrassed to buy a packet of condoms and both she and her partner imagine that she is too old to get pregnant.

STERILIZATION

Although sterilization can be reversed, it should be regarded as irreversible. Deciding to be sterilized is, therefore, a big decision which should only be taken after considerable thought and discussion with your doctors and partner.

Of a woman. The gynaecologist makes a small cut in her abdomen and then cuts or removes parts of both Fallopian tubes and seals them. The procedure is quick and involves a very short hospital stay. The operation is usually effective but difficult to reverse. Because it does not involve the removal of any hormone-producing organs it does not affect feelings, body or sexual drive at all. Since an egg may be waiting in the womb, a woman should take her usual precautions until she has a menstrual period.

Of a man. Known as a vasectomy, this operation is very simple. Using a local anaesthetic, the surgeon closes the tube down which sperm travel from the testes to the penis. Afterwards, although there are no sperm in the semen, there is no visible difference and no other effects. It usually takes ten or twenty ejaculations to get rid of waiting sperm and men are usually advised to have two tests done to make sure that their semen is free of sperm. Reversing the operation is very difficult, but possible.

'MORNING AFTER' PILLS

Doctors can prescribe pills which prevent implantation should an egg have been fertilized. These pills need to be taken within, at most, seventy-two hours of making love. The pills seem safe and effective.

THE ABORTION PILL

This is a new pill which can bring about an abortion, if it is taken within a few weeks of a pregnancy beginning.

CHAPTER NINE

Sexually Transmitted Diseases

Anyone who has sex is, theoretically at least, exposed to the risk of contracting a sexually transmitted disease. There are about twenty-five different specific diseases which can be transmitted through sex (though if you wanted to count all the diseases that could be transmitted during intercourse you would have to include diseases such as tuberculosis, influenza, chicken pox and measles).

PROTECTION

The only way to avoid the risk of contracting a sexually transmitted disease is either to avoid sex completely, to make sure that you only ever have sex with virgins or to remain totally faithful to someone who remains totally faithful to you.

A less certain way to protect yourself and to minimize your risk of contracting an unwanted disease is to make sure that you always use some form of mechanical contraception (preferably a condom), to pass urine immediately after sex (that helps by washing away some potential infections) and (also immediately after sex) to wash yourself with soap and water.

If you have ANY symptoms of a sexually transmitted disease seek medical advice straight away. If you do not have symptoms but suspect that you could have an infection still go for a check up. Most diseases can be dealt with more effectively when treated early.

NOTE

DO TAKE CARE WHEN USING PUBLIC LAVATORIES. IT IS POSSIBLE TO PICK UP SOME SEXUALLY TRANSMITTED DISEASES FROM INFECTED TOILET SEATS.

GONORRHOEA

Still one of the most common sexually transmitted diseases. Of all the women who contract gonorrhoea sixty per cent will have no symptoms at all. The rest will usually notice fairly vague, non-specific symptoms such as a vaginal discharge and a burning sensation on passing urine (the same symptoms as are usually found with chlamydia below). The symptoms of gonorrhoea usually develop within two to ten days of having sex with an infected partner.

Diagnosing and treating gonorrhoea is important because the disease can cause pelvic infections and sometimes results in sterility in women. In addition if a woman with gonorrhoea gives birth her baby can contract an extremely unpleasant eye infection.

CHLAMYDIA

Although it was virtually unheard of just a few years ago chlamydia is now reputed to be the commonest sexually transmitted disease in the western world. It is a common cause of problems among new-born babies and leads to sterility in thousands of women every year. It is also believed to cause approximately fifty per cent of all cases of female pelvic inflammatory disease.

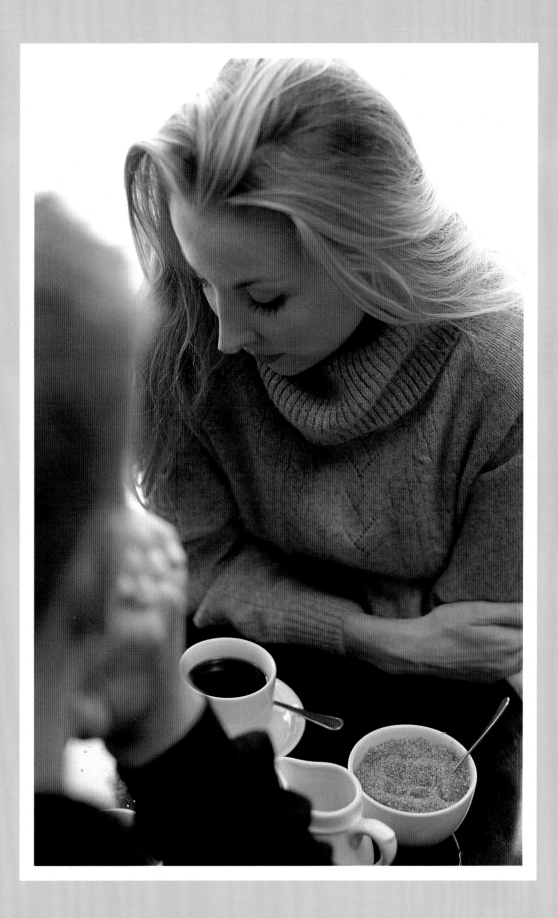

The importance of chlamydia only became apparent when researchers investigated the condition known as non-specific urethritis (also known as NSU and non-gonococcal urethritis) and found that in about half the cases they looked at the organism responsible was in fact chlamydia. Non-specific genital infection is also likely to be caused by chlamydia.

The symptoms of chlamydia mean that it is often mistaken for gonorrhoea. Women who have the disease often have pain on passing urine and a vaginal discharge. Men get similar symptoms: burning on passing urine and a discharge.

The difference between chlamydia and gonorrhoea is that when penicillin is given chlamydia infections do not clear up. Other drugs such as tetracycline or erythromycin are needed to control chlamydia.

GENITAL WARTS

The incidence of genital warts is increasing. Like all warts these are caused by a virus. Transmitted by sexual contact, genital warts can be found on the penis, around the outside of the vagina and elsewhere in the immediate area of the genitals. Sometimes there may be only one or two small warts visible but occasionally huge warty growths can develop.

Genital warts can be burnt off, frozen off, removed surgically or painted with caustic substances, but all these treatments *must* be applied by a doctor.

HERPES

Herpes is not a new disease (though from the publicity it has had in the last decade or so you might imagine that it was). The Roman emperor Tiberius tried to stamp it out by banning kissing and William Shakespeare wrote about it in his play *Romeo and Juliet*.

There are two types of herpes – herpes simplex 1 (HSV1) and herpes simplex 2 (HSV2) – but there are many different strains of the viruses. Both types of virus can infect either the mouth or the genital area and, although herpes can be transmitted sexually it can also be transmitted in other ways. It is possible to get herpes more than once, because of the existence of different types of virus.

The first symptoms of a herpes infection can appear up to thirty years after the virus first arrived on the skin. An infected mother washing her child can give it herpes which does not erupt until half a lifetime later. The herpes HSV2 can live for seventy-two hours on towels, clothing and lavatory seats.

Although it does not get as much publicity as it used to herpes is still increasing very rapidly. Ironically the increase is at least partly due to improving social conditions. A generation or two ago most people acquired immunity to herpes when they were exposed to the infection as children, but these days we rarely share baths or towels with one another and so we grow up without ever being exposed to the herpes viruses. As a result we do not develop any immunity to them and are therefore far more vulnerable when we reach adulthood.

Babies are the other group of people most at risk. Herpes is said to kill about one baby in every 250,000 in the western world, with half of those babies acquiring the infection from their mothers and the other half from visitors or nurses. If a pregnant woman has active herpes the danger can be minimized by delivering her baby by Caesarian section.

The first symptoms of herpes usually appear gradually. A few days, perhaps a week after sexual contact with someone carrying the infection, the sufferer will feel a little tired. He or she may suffer from flu-like symptoms such as fever, headache, stiffness and backache. As these general symptoms develop so more specific symptoms will appear. There will be some local genital irritation and very probably a discharge. There may also be pain or a burning sensation when urine is passed. About four days or so after the onset of the irritation small blisters will probably appear on the penis or around the vagina and these may well be extremely sore.

The glands in the groin will usually swell too.

Severe recurrences of herpes are relatively rare and around a third of sufferers have just one attack and no more. Another third of sufferers get occasional, infrequent and relatively minor outbreaks. Only a third of herpes sufferers get troublesome recurrences – and these are usually less painful than the initial attacks.

THINGS TO REMEMBER ABOUT HERPES

1. You should avoid having sex whenever a herpes lesion is visible.

2. You must wash your hands carefully after visiting the toilet.

3. Don't sit on the seats in public lavatories.

4. Be gentle during sex if you have herpes: trauma can bring back symptoms.

5. Use plenty of lubrication during sex to keep friction to a minimum.

6. A condom will provide some protection, as will barrier creams.

7. You must not kiss or touch cold sores or genital sores.

8. Remember that stress and anxiety can make herpes lesions worse.

THRUSH

The proper name is candidiasis although thrush is also known as moniliasis. Tens of thousands of women get it for the first time every week. Hundreds of thousands are long-term sufferers. Although it isn't necessarily transmitted by sex (the fungus that causes it can just start to grow) thrush is nonetheless one of the most common sexually transmitted diseases around.

The bug that causes the infection is not particularly rare. Most people have the *candida albicans* fungus living on their skin or somewhere else in their bodies. But when the fungus starts to grow out of control problems occur. Theoretically the candida fungus can grow almost anywhere but like most fungi the infection that causes thrush prefers somewhere soft, moist, warm and dark. And that means that the vagina is the place most likely to be targeted.

The first symptom of thrush is usually a white, itchy discharge. Sex becomes painful, uncomfortable and unpleasant and the itching can be unbearable. Thick, white patches often appear around the outside of the vagina. The chances of a candida fungal infection developing are increased when the naturally rather warm and moist area of the vagina is made unnaturally more so. Wearing nylon underwear, tights or close-fitting trousers all make it easier for the candida fungus to grow.

But it isn't only what you wear that determines your susceptibility to thrush.

• The change in circulating oestrogens that occurs during pregnancy or when a woman takes the contraceptive pill can also encourage thrush to develop.

• Eating too much sugar makes the environment even better.

• Being overweight means that fatty folds around the outside of the vagina keep the area unusually moist and warm.

• Taking antibiotics upsets the natural balance of bugs and makes thrush more likely.

• Scratches and skin abrasions can also increase the likelihood of thrush developing.

• Inserting a tampon with dirty hands can put up your chances of developing the infection.

There are a number of things you can do to reduce your chances of contracting thrush – or to increase your chances of getting rid of it.

Good local hygiene is important but it is not necessary to use antiseptics or deodorants; indeed, such products can increase your problems by irritating the area. Skirts, stockings and no underwear are much better for keeping the area well 'aired'.

If a candida infection develops, visit your doctor who may prescribe an antifungal cream or pessaries. The doctor may also want your partner to have a course of treatment since the candida infection can be passed between the two of you during sex.

Some women have reported a reduction in

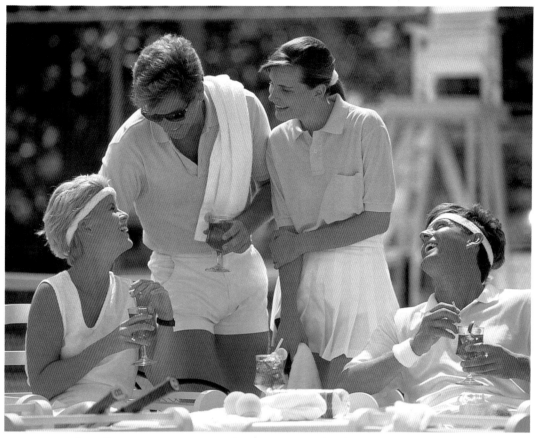

symptoms after dipping tampons in plain yoghurt and inserting them. Yoghurt contains the lactobacilli bacteria which compete with and often oust the infection.

SYPHILIS

Although in the 19th and early 20th centuries syphilis used to be the most feared of all sexually transmitted diseases it is now relatively rare.

It usually begins with a painless sore that looks rather like an ulcer and which usually appears on the penis or the outside of the vagina. The patient will probably also have a flu-like illness – together with swollen glands. The first symptoms of syphilis usually appear anything from nine to ninety days after having sex with an infected partner.

If caught early syphilis can be treated effectively with antibiotics. Even if left untreated the symptoms disappear spontaneously after a few weeks or months, and sufferers usually stop being infectious about two years after first con-

tracting the disease (although mothers can still pass the disease onto their babies after that).

The real danger is that if syphilis goes untreated it can produce heart or brain disease twenty or thirty years later. It is this which makes syphilis one of the most horrifying of all the sexually transmitted diseases.

TRICHOMONAS

Since it produces a nasty vaginal discharge trichomonas is sometimes confused with thrush. The difference is that the discharge associated with trichomonas is usually yellowish green and invariably smells. There is normally some redness and soreness around the vagina too. Trichomonas, like thrush, means that sexual intercourse is extremely sore and uncomfortable. Although trichomonas is commonly transmitted through sex, it can be picked up from infected towels and lavatory seats. If you think you could have this – or any other vaginal infection – see your doctor for the appropriate treatment.

AIDS

WHAT DO AIDS AND HIV STAND FOR?

AIDS and HIV are not the same thing.

AIDS stands for

'Auto Immune Deficiency Syndrome'.

HIV stands for

'Human Immunodeficiency Virus'.

The Human Immunodeficiency Virus, which can be transmitted from one person to another, can remain dormant with no outward signs of illness inside an infected individual for a long time before producing any symptoms.

Inside the body the virus affects lymphocytes and monocytes - types of cells which play a vital role in the mechanism the body uses to defend itself against infection.

If an individual has become infected with the Human Immunodeficiency Virus he or she is said to be HIV positive.

When the virus has affected the body, diminishing its ability to protect itself against infection, the individual is said to have AIDS .

The main AIDS controversy concerns the ways in which the virus can be passed from one individual to another. Contrary to popular rumour the virus is quite difficult to catch, and is usually transmitted when the blood of an infected individual mixes with the blood of someone who hasn't got the disease.

WHAT ARE THE SYMPTOMS OF AIDS?

Doctors first became aware of the effects of this virus in the early 1980s in America when they saw a number of young male homosexuals suffering from a rare form of skin cancer called Kaposi's sarcoma and an unusual respiratory infection. All the patients had damaged immune systems – in other words their bodies were not able to fight disease well.

The first physical signs of AIDS developing are swollen glands, under the jaw, in the groin, armpit and neck. Since these symptoms are fre-quently found with many other much commoner diseases, this is not a sure sign of AIDS. The patient usually only finds out that he (or she) is infected with the virus if he has a blood test later on, which shows that his body has started to develop antibodies to the Human Immunodeficiency Virus 1 (HIV was first identified in France in 1983).

After the gland swelling patients get a variety of minor infections and symptoms such as weight loss, fever, diarrhoea, thrush and dermatitis which can prove difficult to shake off.

In the final stage of AIDS - contracted by half of all people infected with HIV within eight years - a whole host of illnesses develop because of the body's inability to fight off infections and cancers. People who have used drugs or alcohol or who have poor health may be more vulnerable to the disease.

The most common serious problems are pneumonia (a threatening chest infection), the type of skin tumour (Kaposi's sarcoma) which affected the first victims of AIDS, and some types of brain disease which cause paralysis, dementia and blindness. It is often possible to slow down the specific disorders which develop, but because the body cannot help itself a cure is not possible. Treatment becomes increasingly difficult as the disease progresses, and indeed is a matter of providing nursing care as much as medical care. In the final stages the patient will develop endless coughs and chest infections and may acquire more than one type of cancer.

THE ONE SEXUAL PRACTICE EVERYONE SHOULD AVOID

If governments had warned people of the hazards associated with anal sex the incidence of AIDS would have been far smaller. Although anal sex is illegal in many parts of the world, it is remarkably popular among heterosexuals as well as homosexuals. One of the world's biggest sex surveys showed that as many as one in ten heterosexual couples regularly have anal sex.

Way back in 1987 doctors knew the sexual

practice most likely to lead to HIV and AIDS virus infection was receptive anal intercourse. A survey involving more than one thousand heterosexual, homosexual and bisexual men, showed that 'receptive anal genital contact is the major mode of HIV infection'. The study found that almost half the homosexuals and bisexuals tested positive for HIV but no heterosexual men were positive. The report went on to conclude that 'there was no evidence of epidemic spread due to any other mode of transmission'.

This report made sense when I first read it. After all, the evidence showed that AIDS was primarily a blood borne disease and, whereas ordinary vaginal sex does not usually lead to damaged tissues (and therefore bleeding) anal sex often does.

Then, in 1988 the *British Medical Journal* published a paper on 'The heterosexual transmission of HIV by haemophiliacs'. Doctors had studied 13 haemophiliacs and their partners for three years. Their conclusion was 'in the absence of other risk factors transmission of HIV from men to women by vaginal intercourse is infrequent'. A study carried out on women attending genitourinary clinics in London revealed that more than half of the 424 women who said that they had non regular sexual partners never used a condom. The two women who were HIV positive who completed a questionnaire on their sexual behaviour reported that they had experienced anal sex.

One of the most important papers published on the subject of AIDS was probably the one produced in 1989 on AIDS in Paris by the European Study Group, co-ordinated by the World Health Organization Collaborating Centre. It concluded, after an international survey, that: 'the only sexual practice that clearly increased the risk of male to female transmission of AIDS was anal intercourse'. They also stated

"Wearing a condom provides a certain amount of protection and avoiding anal sex is essential if you want to keep your chances of contracting AIDS to a minimum."

that: 'no other sexual practices have been associated with the risk of transmission.'

In the 1980s, the incidence of AIDS rose dramatically as it spread among homosexuals and heterosexuals practising anal sex. For a variety of reasons (some religious, some political, and some simply commercial) horrendous and absurd forecasts were made about the future.

But by the early 1990s, the number of people who were in the high risk categories (heterosexuals and homosexuals who practised anal sex and who also had more than one partner) and who had not contracted the disease - and were, therefore, considered vulnerable to it - had fallen. Inevitably the incidence of the disease started to fall.

The British Institute of Actuaries (the job of actuaries is to give insurance companies their advice on risks) has stated that there is 'no evidence to support the hypothesis of a "heterosexual explosion" of AIDS or HIV infection in this country' and the International AIDS Coordinator at the National Cancer Institute in the United States of America has announced that 'the HIV epidemic in North America and Europe probably peaked...in the mid 1980s'.

I have looked for independent scientific evidence supporting those who claim that AIDS constitutes a major threat to all heterosexuals, but I am afraid I have been unable to find anything which convinces me.

Many of those who still argue that AIDS is a major threat to heterosexuals point to Africa, where AIDS is much more common among heterosexuals. Even if we leave aside the question of whether or not the African virus is the same one, and the controversy over immune systems and susceptibilities, there are a number of simple explanations for this phenomenon.

First, other sexually transmitted diseases which produce bleeding sores are common, and frequently untreated, in Africa. It is, therefore, much easier for blood to spread from one individual to another. And second, anal sex is widely used as a form of contraception.

Anal sex is, of course, also extremely popular among male homosexuals, and it is for this reason that AIDS has spread to such an extent among homosexual men.

It seems to me that we are all at risk of contracting HIV and AIDS - although for most of us the risks are relatively slight. However, the independent evidence currently available seems to show that two activities in particular, practising anal sex and sharing hypodermic needles, are especially likely to lead to the spread of AIDS.

It seems a pity that governments still have not managed to get the message across that it is anal sex that people should avoid 'like the plague', especially if they have casual sex and several partners. Since 1987 it has been abundantly clear that anal sex is a sexual practice everyone should avoid.

How to Avoid AIDS

Wearing a condom provides a certain amount of protection and avoiding anal sex is essential if you want to keep your chances of contracting AIDS to a minimum.

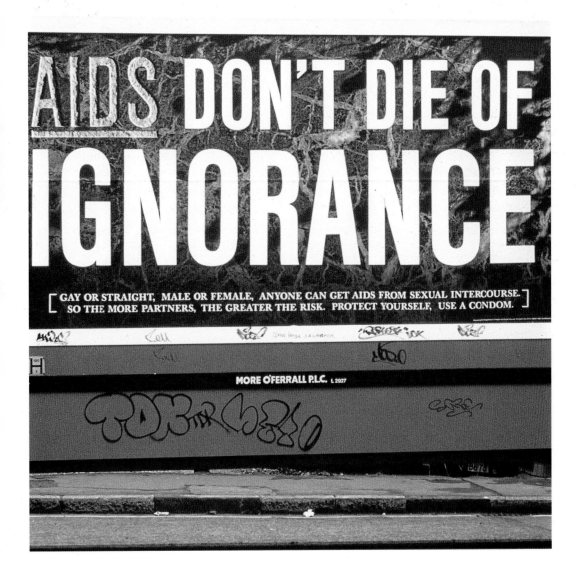

CHAPTER TEN

Your Top 100 Questions About Sex

Q **IS IT POSSIBLE FOR ME TO CHOOSE THE SEX OF MY BABY?**

A Over the centuries many people have tried to find ways to manipulate the odds and to choose the sex of their baby. The ancient Greeks believed that sperm from the left testicle meant that a girl would be born, while sperm from the right testicle would produce a boy. In order to try to choose the sex of their next baby, Greek fathers would have one testicle temporarily tied off. In Austria women giving birth who wanted a son the next time, would ask the midwife to bury the placenta or afterbirth underneath the nearest nut tree.

Women living on the Pelew Islands, east of the Philippines in the Pacific Ocean, used to dress up in their partner's clothes in the belief that this would help ensure that they would give birth to a baby boy.

Popular theories seem to emerge all over the world. One modern idea popular in several countries is that if a man wants a boy, he should make sure that he throws his underpants down on the right hand side of the bed, before making love to his partner.

Other rather bizarre but widespread theories designed to ensure the birth of a baby boy include making love with your shoes on, eating a raw egg beforehand or making love only when the wind is coming from the north.

These days scientists try to be more logical when advising parents on the best ways to choose the sex of their babies. Here is a summary of the best available information:

1. If you want a boy, make love on the day of ovulation. If you want a girl, make love at least two days before ovulation – success is not guaranteed of course. For information on ovulation see page 92.

2. If you want a girl wait until you are older. Young couples seem to have more sons, while older parents seem to be more likely to give birth to daughters.

3. If you want a boy make love during a war. There is a rise in the number of boys born during or just after a war!

4. If you have a string of sons and are desperate for a daughter keep trying – the odds get better. The more children you have the more likely you are to have a girl.

5. Women who want a girl should either marry an anaesthetist or a fighter pilot. Both groups seem to father more girls than boys.

6. Eat plenty of fish (but no shellfish), lots of vegetables (but no lettuce, raw cabbage or cauliflower, spinach or cress) and lots of fresh fruit if you want a boy. If you want a girl keep your consumption of salt low but drink plenty of milk and eat lots of rice and pasta.

Q **IF YOU HAVE SEX FOR TOO LONG CAN IT DO YOU ANY DAMAGE?**

A Neither the penis nor the vagina are designed for long periods of use. Too much rubbing of the penis will eventually make it sore and may cause a burning sensation when urine is passed. Women can suffer from a sore and itchy vagina or the unpleasant symptoms of cystitis.

Q Is LOSING YOUR VIRGINITY ALWAYS A PAINFUL EXPERIENCE?

A No. Apprehension and anxiety may produce some vaginismus (see page 70) but if your partner is gentle losing your virginity should not be a painful experience.

Q Is THERE ANY DIFFERENCE BETWEEN A CLITORAL AND A VAGINAL ORGASM?

A Sigmund Freud argued that little girls discover that they can achieve orgasm by stimulating the clitoris and later find that they must transfer their sexual response from the clitoris to the vagina. He claimed that women who fail to do this become vaginally frigid even though they can masturbate themselves to orgasm. He was wrong. During intercourse the thrusting of the penis causes the labia minora to move and stimulate the clitoris. The clitoris can, therefore, participate in ordinary vaginal intercourse. There is only one type of orgasm and it doesn't matter what is stimulated – the clitoris, the vagina, the breasts or the anus.

Q Does EXERCISE REDUCE OR INCREASE YOUR APPETITE FOR SEX?

A Regular exercise makes it easier for women and men to become sexually aroused and makes them better lovers. People who exercise regularly say that their desire for sex increases and that they have more confidence in bed.

Q WHAT HAPPENS DURING MALE CIRCUMCISION? AND WHY IS IT DONE?

A In male circumcision the foreskin which normally covers the glans of the penis is

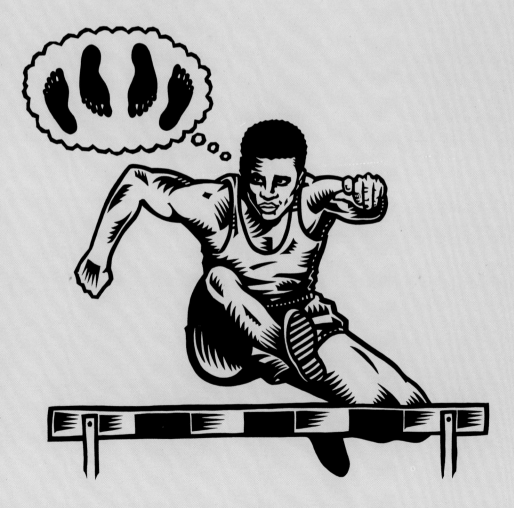

removed. About half the male population is circumcised these days. Sometimes this is done for religious reasons (for example Jewish boys are circumcised) and sometimes as a routine procedure because some doctors believe that a circumcised penis is more hygenic. It is certainly true that if a foreskin is too tight it can hinder normal erection, while dead skin, dirt and stale fluids can accumulate underneath it and become infected. One side effect of circumcision is that it makes the glans of the penis more dry and less sensitive – this usually means that ejaculation is delayed a little during intercourse. However, as long as the organ is clean most women don't seem to mind, though some prefer one style and some the other.

Q I HAVE HEARD THAT ALCOHOL CAN BE AN APHRODISIAC, BUT I THOUGHT THAT ALCOHOL CAUSED IMPOTENCE.

A In large quantities alcohol may increase desire but diminish performance. It certainly can cause impotence in men and frigidity in women. If taken in small quantities, alcohol can be an aphrodisiac, releasing inhibitions and suppressing fears and anxieties. Alcohol works as an aphrodisiac in two ways. It depresses the restrictive control centres in the brain and thereby allows desires which are normally suppressed to surface. In addition it causes a general dilatation of the body's superficial blood vessels and produces a generalized skin glow.

Q WHY ARE WOMEN CIRCUMCISED?

A For religious or cultural reasons. There are no medical reasons. The operation may involve the removal of one or more of these: the clitoris, the clitoral hood, the labia minora and the labia majora. The consequences include bleeding, infection and a host of sexual problems. When female circumcision was first carried out in Arabia and Africa the aim was to reduce a woman's sex drive and to stop her straying from her husband or masturbating. Unfortunately it is still common practice in some countries.

Q IS IT TRUE THAT MARIJUANA IS AN APHRODISIAC?

A It removes inhibitions (in the same way that alcohol does) but has no direct, stimulating sexual effect. Indeed, some evidence suggests that marijuana may lower the amount of circulating testosterone.

Q DOES VITAMIN B CURE IMPOTENCE?

A I don't think so. See page 64 for advice on curing impotence.

Q IS IT TRUE THAT VITAMIN E INCREASES SEXUAL DESIRE AND IMPROVES SEXUAL PERFORMANCE?

A Vitamin E originally earned its massive reputation as an aphrodisiac on the basis of a limited amount of research work done on rat fertility patterns. I have been unable to find any clinical evidence to prove that humans can improve their sexual prowess or performance by taking vitamin E.

Q IS CHOCOLATE AN APHRODISIAC?

A Since the nineteenth century, chocolate has been regarded as a sexual stimulant and given as a love token. Chocolate contains a chemical called phenylethylamine, a substance related to the amphetamines, which is the 'love chemical' which helps us fall in love.

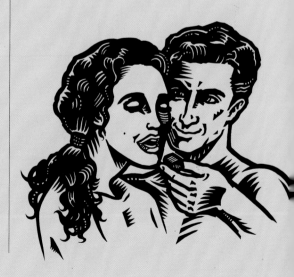

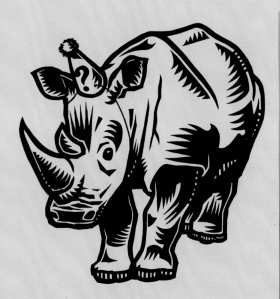

thought and can produce terrifying results. Psilocybe has far less dramatic sexual effects but has a chemical structure quite similar to that of LSD and is, therefore, a hallucinogenic drug.

Q ARE MINERALS SUCH AS ZINC AND IRON LIKELY TO IMPROVE SEXUAL PERFORMANCE?
A Not unless your diet is deficient in minerals. In which case it would be far more sensible to improve your diet.

Q WHAT ARE PHEROMONES?
A Both men and women produce chemical substances called pheromones which are designed to arouse and stimulate members of the opposite sex and these can be far more stimulating than artificial perfumes. The smells associated with the secretions produced by the vaginas of non-ovulating women are far less attractive to men than the smells produced by secretions during ovulation. The production of pheromones is designed to attract men to women at a time when the women are most likely to conceive. If a group of men gather round one woman at a party then it may be that she is ovulating. In order to make the best of your pheromones you should bathe several hours before meeting someone you want to attract in order to remove unpleasant odours and allow the smells of your pheromones to break through.

Q WHY IS POWDERED RHINOCEROS HORN AN APHRODISIAC?
A It isn't. But it acquired its reputation as an aphrodisiac because of its phallic shape.

Q IS AMYL NITRATE AN APHRODISIAC?
A Amyl nitrate increases the blood supply to various parts of the body and can make an individual feel more excited, but there are real dangers with this substance and it is not safe for use as an aphrodisiac. Some users claim that if you break an ampoule of amyl nitrate and inhale the fumes, you will feel a rush of sexual excitement. It is also claimed that the drug helps to relax the anal sphincter (making it popular with homosexuals and heterosexuals wanting to try anal sex) but the hazards of taking this drug far outweigh any value.

Q IS IT NORMAL FOR ONE PARTNER TO HAVE TO HELP TO PUT THE PENIS INTO THE VAGINA? OR SHOULD IT FIND ITS OWN WAY THERE WITHOUT ANY HELP?
A It is quite normal for the penis to need a little help.

Q ARE 'MAGIC MUSHROOMS' EFFECTIVE APHRODISIACS?
A Psilocybe and amanita, obtained from two mushrooms with alleged sexual power, are used separately or together. Amanita is said to give great energy and staying power. Some experimenters have reported that it produces forceful and unnaturally prolonged orgasms with repeated ejaculations and violent vaginal contractions. It also distorts the processes of

Q WHAT IS THE BEST APHRODISIAC?
A Probably clothes. Many men are turned on by black stockings, high-heeled shoes, uplift bras, garter belts, skin-tight trousers and sweaters, low-cut dresses, flimsy nightwear and so on. And most women are turned on by the knowledge that they are turning men on.

Q Is ginseng an aphrodisiac?

A Ginseng gained its reputation because of its phallic shaped root, but the evidence does not support its reputation.

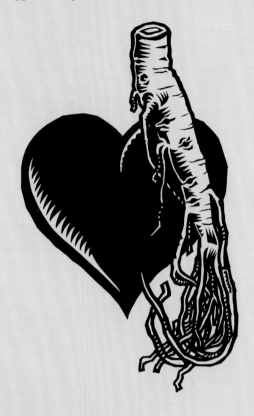

Q Do any prescribed drugs have an effect on sexual behaviour?

A Yes. Some prescribed drugs can produce impotence (see page 64). It is reputed that other prescribed drugs may increase sexual appetite. One doctor has reported that a forty-year-old woman took an appetite suppressant and found that her sexual appetite rose so much that her husband had to take another job nearer to home, so that he could call in at lunchtime to satisfy his wife's greatly increased sexual demands.

Q Why do some people shout out during sex?

A People who are demonstrative often make loud sounds during sex. They may cry, groan, scream, sob, grunt, moan or whimper. Some people shout out fairly obvious things like: 'I'm coming!' Some yell out 'No' when that is clearly the last thing that they mean. Some blaspheme. Some shout the name of a previous lover (embarrassing and potentially expensive). People who make a noise find it difficult to stop but others may be embarrassed, particularly if the room has thin walls. As a general rule men and women who make a noise during sex reach an orgasm more quickly, but just because people are silent during sex it doesn't meant that they are not enjoying themselves. Finally, if you enjoy oral sex remember that it is rude to speak with your mouth full!

Q Which foods are aphrodisiacs?

A Figs have a sexy reputation because some people think they look like the vulva of a woman. Cucumbers, bananas, carrots and other similarly shaped foods gain their reputation because of their phallic shape. The avocado pear has a reputation as an aphrodisiac because it is the same sort of shape as a woman's womb. (The Aztecs had such a high regard for the aphrodisiac qualities of the avocado that they kept all their virgins indoors during the avocado season). Some foods have a sexy reputation because of their smell. So, foods with a 'musky' odour such as asparagus, artichokes, truffles and mushrooms are regarded as aphrodisiacs. The long established association between oysters and sex is

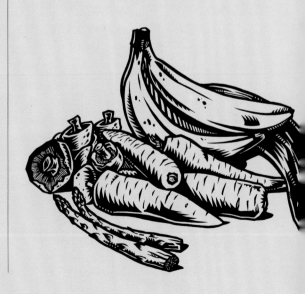

difficult to explain, although oysters do contain chemicals related to sex hormones; some users claim that the opening oyster shell reminds them of a woman.

Q WHY DO SO MANY OLDER WOMEN LIKE YOUNGER MEN?

A Younger men are more virile and often look more attractive. Women like young men for the same reason that older men chase young girls. It makes sound physiological sense for older women to like younger men. Older women are often at their sexual peak long after older men have started on the downhill slide. Women reach a peak in their thirties and forties. Men reach their sexual peak in their late teens and early twenties. Young men like older women because they are more experienced, more skilled, less restrained and often less troublesome.

Q IS IT TRUE THAT SOME WOMEN PASS OUT DURING OR IMMEDIATELY AFTER SEX?

A Yes. It is called the 'little death'. It happens to women more than men. Some individuals have a sort of semi-fit. Others just drift into unconsciousness. It can be scary for the partner staying awake. If you pass out regularly it is sensible to warn new partners beforehand. Otherwise you might come to in an ambulance.

Q IS IT TRUE THAT IF YOU DON'T HAVE SEX FOR A LONG WHILE YOUR SEX DRIVE WILL START TO DISAPPEAR?

A Yes. Regular sex keeps the level of testosterone up. If sexual activity decreases then testosterone production falls. If you don't use it you will lose it. If you don't have a partner you can keep in training with regular bouts of masturbation. It can take a couple of months to recover a lost sex drive.

Q CAN A WOMAN RAPE A MAN?

A Technically, yes. But legally the courts do not seem to take male rape very seriously if it is performed by a woman.

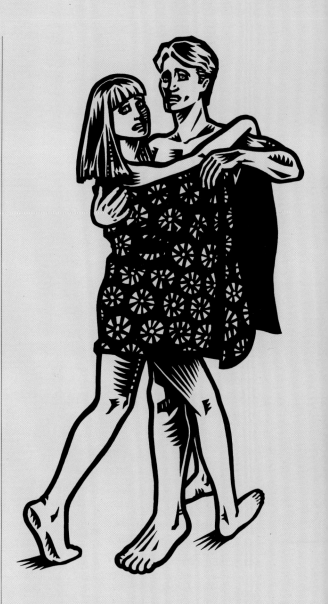

Q CAN A PENIS EVER GET STUCK IN A VAGINA?

A It depends on what you mean by 'stuck'. It is possible for vaginal muscles to go into spasm or for a vagina to contract before the penis shrinks but these problems are short-lived. Those stories about men and women shuffling into the local hospital with a blanket wrapped around them are apocryphal.

Q HOW LONG SHOULD SEX LAST?

A How long is a good holiday? If you are both panting for sexual release good sex may last two minutes. If you have just met then good sex can last all night and all the next day.

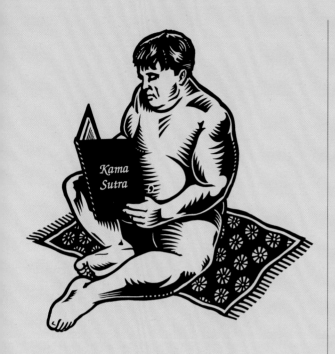

Q Does weight have any significant effect on sexual prowess?

A If you are vastly overweight then you will probably feel embarrassed about undressing and you may find many sexual positions uncomfortable or impossible. But being too thin isn't sexy either. For example, surveys repeatedly show that most men prefer their partners to be curvaceous and slightly on the 'plump' side rather than thin.

Q Is it true that men don't need foreplay?

A No. Men need and enjoy foreplay just as much as women. Many cases of impotence could be prevented by good foreplay. It helps to build up a good, firm erection and to prepare the penis for sex. The better the foreplay the better the sex and the better the orgasm.

Q Why are women often at their sexiest when it is most inconvenient — that is, during a menstrual period?

A Most human emotions go in cycles and the sex drive is no exception. The few days before a period are, for over a third of all women, the sexiest time of the month. The next sexiest time is the days during and immediately after she has had her period.

Q Shouldn't a woman's nipples get erect when she is aroused sexually?

A Some do and some don't. Nipple erection is an entirely involuntary response. Small muscle fibres within the nipple contract when stimulated in certain ways (cold and touch are two common stimulants) and that makes the nipple stand up. But if nipples are very small they may not have the facility to become erect. And if they are very large then it may not be noticeable when they become erect. If you really want to find out what a particular nipple looks like when it is fully erect, you could try splashing it with cold water. (But if you do this to someone else's nipple, I suggest that you get their permission first.)

Q My boyfriend always gets a rash on his penis after I perform oral sex on him. Can you explain this?

A He is probably allergic to your lipstick. Change your brand or try removing your lipstick before you make love.

Q Is it true that women can sometimes become allergic to semen?

A Yes. But this is rare. When it happens one answer is for the man to use a condom.

Q How much semen does the average man produce in one ejaculate?

A About a teaspoonful.

Q How will I know if I have an orgasm?

A You MAY have a mind-blowing, earth-shattering experience that threatens to blow the top off your head. But you are more likely to get a pleasant physical sensation, a feeling of warmth and a bit of a 'buzz' around your genital area. Afterwards you will probably feel rather relaxed and sleepy. Men don't usually have any difficulty in telling when they have come. Women who are expecting something out of this world may not realize that the rather nice feeling they get is an orgasm.

Q CAN SOME WOMEN HAVE MULTIPLE ORGASMS?

A After men have ejaculated there is a period during which they cannot have an erection. This period may last for a few minutes or for an hour or more. This doesn't happen to women. If properly stimulated some women can have a whole series of orgasms – one after the other. The vibrator has revolutionized the female orgasm. With a vibrator a woman may be able to have dozens of orgasms in one session, stopping only when she is totally exhausted.

Q HOW LONG DOES IT TAKE THE AVERAGE WOMAN TO REACH AN ORGASM?

A That's a bit like asking 'What is the bust size of the average woman?'. If a woman is going to reach an orgasm through straight intercourse then ten minutes of foreplay followed by five minutes of vigorous sex should be long enough. Many women need manual stimulation in addition to vaginal penetration before they can have an orgasm. For them eight hours of continuous thrusting would not be enough to produce an orgasm.

Q ONE OF MY BREASTS IS SLIGHTLY LARGER THAN THE OTHER. IT IS VERY EMBARRASSING. IS IT UNUSUAL? CAN ANYTHING BE DONE ABOUT IT?

A Most women have breasts of slightly different sizes. If the difference is noticeable (if you can't find a bra to fit comfortably) or embarrassing, arrange to see a plastic surgeon.

Q I HAD A HYSTERECTOMY TWO YEARS AGO. DO I STILL NEED TO HAVE REGULAR CERVICAL SMEARS DONE?

A That depends entirely upon whether or not the surgeon performing your operation removed the *whole* of your uterus (a total hysterectomy) or just part of it (a partial hysterectomy). If you had a total hysterectomy you don't have a cervix left, so you can't have a cervical smear. But if the surgeon only removed part of your uterus or womb you could have a cervix left. Your own doctor should be able to tell you exactly what was done and whether you still need smears.

Q IS IT TRUE THAT THE PHYSIOLOGY OF A SNEEZE IS THE SAME AS THE PHYSIOLOGY OF AN ORGASM?

A No. And I suggest that you avoid the temptation to say 'God bless you' next time your partner climaxes.

Q WHAT IS A BISEXUAL?

A Someone who can enjoy sex with members of either sex.

Q I SUFFER TERRIBLY FROM THE PRE-MENSTRUAL SYNDROME FOR TWO WEEKS EVERY MONTH. MY BREASTS SWELL AND BECOME PAINFUL AND MY ANKLES SWELL UP TOO. I ALSO GET VERY DEPRESSED AND TEARFUL.

A Eat regular meals to keep your blood sugar levels up. Avoid salt, caffeine and alcohol during the days before a period. And talk to your doctor who may be able to prescribe a course of useful hormone treatment.

Q I AM 47 YEARS OLD. SINCE MY PERIODS STOPPED SIX MONTHS AGO I HAVE BEEN VERY MISERABLE. I GET NIGHT SWEATS AND I FLUSH A LOT. CAN YOU RECOMMEND ANYTHING?

A Ask your doctor if you are a suitable candidate for Hormone Replacement Therapy. It can work wonders for the symptoms you have, though your doctor may be unwilling to prescribe it if you have a personal or family history of heart disease, liver trouble or cancer.

Q I PUT ON A LOT OF WEIGHT WHEN I WAS PREGNANT LAST YEAR. IT LEFT ME WITH TERRIBLE STRETCH MARKS. IS THERE ANYTHING

I CAN DO ABOUT THEM?

A Your local pharmacist should be able to recommend a suitable camouflage cream. I don't recommend plastic surgery for stretch marks: the result can be scars that are more noticeable than the stretch marks. Remember that although stretch marks rarely disappear entirely, they do usually fade with time.

Q MY DOCTOR HAS DIAGNOSED FIBROIDS AND HAS RECOMMENDED THAT I SEE A HOSPITAL SPECIALIST WITH A VIEW TO HAVING A HYSTERECTOMY. IF THIS IS NECESSARY WILL IT MEAN THAT I HAVE AN EARLY MENOPAUSE?

A No. It is extremely unlikely. The menopause develops when hormone production drops. A hysterectomy involves the removal of an organ – the uterus – which has no part to play in hormone production. It is only if a hysterectomy is accompanied by ovary removal that the operation leads to an early menopause.

Q MY BREASTS ARE VERY LARGE AND I GET A TERRIBLE RASH UNDERNEATH THEM IN THE SUMMER. WHAT CAN I DO ABOUT IT?

A You are almost certainly suffering from a condition known as 'intertrigo'. Try to keep the area under your breasts as clean and dry as possible and wear a good supporting bra. If, despite this, the rash still appears visit your doctor. You may need to use a steroid cream or an anti-infective cream for a few days.

Q I HAVE A SMALL SWELLING IN MY SCROTUM. IT HASN'T CHANGED MUCH IN TWO MONTHS. DO YOU THINK I SHOULD TELL MY DOCTOR?

A Yes. Most scrotal swellings are harmless, but those which are not can usually be treated effectively if they are found early.

Q IS IT POSSIBLE TO HAVE SEX AFTER A PROSTATE OPERATION?

A Yes. The removal of the prostate gland does not usually have any effect on a man's ability to have sex.

Q MY NIPPLES BECOME VERY SENSITIVE WHEN I AM MAKING LOVE. IS THIS A NORMAL SENSATION FOR A MAN?

A Yes, although the level of sensitivity varies very much from one man to another.

Q MY SON ONLY HAS ONE TESTICLE. HE IS SIX YEARS OLD. IS THERE ANYTHING THAT CAN BE DONE TO BRING THE OTHER TESTICLE DOWN?

A A simple operation should do the trick. And once brought down into its proper place the missing testicle should be able to function perfectly normally.

Q MY HUSBAND-TO-BE HAD A VASECTOMY FOUR YEARS AGO. WE WANT TO HAVE CHILDREN TOGETHER. IS IT POSSIBLE FOR HIM TO HAVE THE VASECTOMY REVERSED?

A Probably. It is a tricky operation but some surgeons will tackle it.

Q I HAVE VERY SMALL BREASTS. WILL I STILL BE ABLE TO BREAST FEED?

A Yes. Your breasts will swell when you have a baby (and will probably remain enlarged afterwards). But even if you cannot produce all the milk your baby needs you should be able to feed him and top up his requirements with a bottle feed.

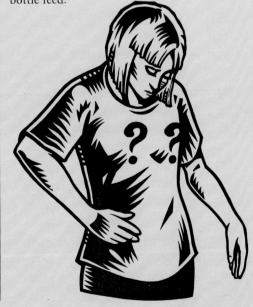

Q My girlfriend was shocked when she found that I am not circumcised. She says that I should get circumcised so that she will be less likely to get cancer. Is this true?

A It is true that some experts believe that women who only sleep with circumcised men are slightly less likely to develop cervical cancer. (And some experts believe that circumcised men are less likely to develop cancer of the penis). But I don't think this is a good argument for having a circumcision. It may be a 'small' operation but there are still risks. You can, I believe, protect yourself and your partner just as well by making sure that you clean the area under your foreskin regularly and thoroughly.

Q I am 19 and have only been to bed with a girl once. It was very embarrassing because I had an orgasm far too soon and she was left very frustrated. She has refused to see me again.

A It is called 'premature ejaculation' and it happens to most men, particularly when they are inexperienced or overexcited. Your girlfriend's behaviour suggests that she is also very inexperienced or just very selfish (or maybe both). See page 65.

Q I've always enjoyed sex but recently I have found it very painful.

A There are numerous possible explanations, but there are 'cures' for nearly all of them. Visit your doctor. A physical examination should enable him to suggest a solution. See page 70.

Q What are the symptoms of a sexually transmitted disease?

A The symptoms vary with the disease (there are around 25 different STDs). But the most common symptoms are: rashes, swellings, urinary symptoms (such as bleeding, frequency and pain), soreness, itching, discharges, lumps, ulcers and warts. Even if you don't have any of these symptoms and you *think* that you could

have a sexually transmitted disease get professional help straight away. All infections are much easier to treat early on, than when they've been given a chance to establish themselves. See pages 104–109.

Q My husband wants to take photographs of me in the nude (only for his personal use, he says). I don't mind (in fact I'm rather excited by the idea) but I'm worried that we might be starting something that could lead to things we'll both regret.

A Stop worrying. One in five women have posed for nude photographs! Make the ground rules clear before you start (eg. no showing the photos to anyone else) and as long as you are both enthusiastic your photo sessions should simply add extra sparkle to your sex life.

Q I have had five children and have been 'stretched' down below rather a lot. Is there an operation I could have to tighten things up a bit?

A Yes. You need to see either a gynaecologist or a plastic surgeon.

Q Is it true that there is a contraceptive pill that can be used after sex?

A Yes. But you need to take it as soon as possible – within a few hours – of having unprotected sex. It is called the 'morning-after' pill (see page 103).

Q Is it possible to get pregnant after having oral sex?

A Yes. If you and your partner do things in the right order, it is theoretically possible. But it's also possible that the baby you have will be the new Messiah. The chances of either event occurring are extremely remote.

Q At what age is it normal to stop having sexual urges? My wife and I are both in our mid-seventies but we still

ENJOY SEX REGULARLY.

A No prizes given I'm afraid. As many as three-quarters of men aged seventy or older still have a regular sex life.

Q IS IT NORMAL FOR PEOPLE TO HAVE SEXUAL FANTASIES?

A Yes. Both men and women have sexual fantasies. Women fantasize more often during sex than men. Both men and women claim that fantasies help them to reach orgasm during as well as outside normal, heterosexual sex. Men and women often feel guilty about their sexual fantasies. But fantasies do not have anything to do with real life.

Q WHY ARE VIBRATORS SO POPULAR?

A The artificial phallus or dildo has been popular for centuries. Sculptures from ancient Babylonia and India show women with dildoes in their hands. Two thousand years ago Greek women used sophisticated dildoes made of leather and fitted with mechanical devices which enabled them to become erect. Modern vibrators are powered by small batteries. Often made in the shape of a penis, they can hasten the onset of an orgasm. They are mostly used by women, who can get great pleasure from using them on or around the clitoris. A woman who has difficulty in reaching an orgasm may find that a vibrator provides her with a welcome release from frustration. If her partner has suffered from feelings of inadequacy he will probably welcome the arrival of the vibrator, which can be an aid to good sex rather than a rival or a threat. Men can enjoy them too, either applied to the penis or around the inside of the anus.

Q IS IT TRUE THAT IF YOU DON'T HAVE SEX REGULARLY YOUR DESIRE WILL EVENTUALLY DISAPPEAR?

A Yes, although once you start a regular sex life again your desire will return. And you can use this answer as an excuse or supporting argument if you like.

Q I WOULD LIKE TO HAVE HAIR ON MY CHEST BECAUSE I THINK IT WOULD HELP TO IMPROVE MY SEX LIFE. CAN YOU RECOMMEND A CREAM I CAN BUY?

A No. I'm afraid there isn't anything. But there are probably as many women who prefer male chests to be hair*less* as there are women who are turned on by hairy chests!

Q WHENEVER WE GO AWAY ON HOLIDAY MY WIFE LIKES TO SUNBATHE TOPLESS. SHE SEEMS TO GET QUITE A THRILL OUT OF EXPOSING HERSELF. IS THIS NORMAL?

A Lots of women enjoy exposing themselves in public, either in the flesh or on photographs (thousands of women who are not professional models allow nude photographs of themselves to be published in magazines). This is quite normal and nothing to worry about.

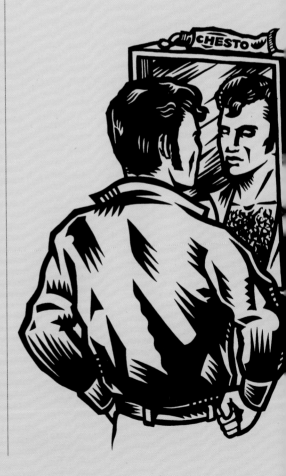

Q WHAT SORT OF THINGS DO MEN FANTASIZE ABOUT?

A When adolescent boys start fantasizing their dreams are largely physical. They fantasize about seducing beautiful women, often mothers of their friends or friends of their mother. A third of all men have fantasies while making love. Here are the most popular male sexual fantasies:

1. Replacing their usual partner with another woman (friend, neighbour, young girl, film star, past lover).
2. Having sex with a woman who resists but finds it so exciting that she gives in.
3. Watching other people have sex.
4. Watching another man (or several men) have sex with their partner.
5. Having group sex.
6. Having a homosexual encounter.
7. Being sexually abused by women.
8. Having sex while an audience watches.
9. Making love in bizarre circumstances.
10. Taking part in a threesome with a man and a woman or two women.
11. Watching a woman have sex with an animal.
12. Watching two women have sex together.
13. Watching a regular partner work as a prostitute.
14. Being raped by a woman.
15. Being spanked.
16. Being involved in food fights with a woman.
17. Being urinated on by a woman.
18. Being a slave to a woman.
19. Being subjected to anal sex by a woman equipped with a large dildo.
20. Having sex with a woman with huge breasts.

Q DO FANTASIES EVER TURN INTO REALITY?

A Sometimes. But not very often. A fantasy is not necessarily a repressed wish. Women sometimes fantasize about being taken forcibly by several men at once. For them the fantasy is entirely different to reality. Similarly, men who fantasize about raping women should not feel guilty; the fantasy is usually a long way from the real thing.

Q WHAT SORT OF THINGS DO WOMEN FANTASIZE ABOUT?

A Female fantasies begin by being more emotional than physical. Girls fantasize about being loved. But in adult life women's fantasies become more physical and are just as explicit as male fantasies. Here are some of the most popular female fantasies.

1. Having sex with a lover in a public place.
2. Being subjected to sex in public.
3. Being exposed in public.
4. Having sex with a stranger.
5. Making love to young boys.
6. Making love to an animal.
7. Being taken by several men at once.
8. Being taken by a stranger from behind – and never seeing his face.
9. Watching others have sex.
10. Having an encounter with a stranger who leaves after sex.
11. Having a lesbian encounter.
12. Stripping on stage.
13. Taking part in a group sexual encounter.
14. Working as a prostitute.
15. Humiliating a man.
16. Being tied down and sexually used by a series of men.
17. Being spanked.
18. Having a male slave.
19. Being forced to perform oral sex on a man.
20. Taking part in a threesome with two men or one man and a woman.

Q I HAVE HEARD THAT SOME WOMEN PIERCE THEIR NIPPLES AND HANG JEWELLERY THROUGH THEM. IS THIS SAFE?

A Nipple piercing has been popular for centuries. In France, in the reign of Louis XIV, the Church condoned the wearing of low-necked dresses as long as the women wearing them had gold rings piercing their exposed nipples. The

Church argued that the gold rings meant that the breasts were not entirely naked. Today, nipple piercing is an increasingly popular fashion. It is also fashionable for some women and men to have their sexual organs pierced and fitted with jewellery. Women sometimes have rings pushed through their labia. The idea is that the weight of the rings will pull down the clitoral hood and stimulate the clitoris. Women also claim that while wearing labial rings their partners are better able to bring them to orgasm. Some men say that they find labial jewellery visually stimulating. It is not uncommon for a man to wear a ring through his foreskin, frenulum, glans or scrotum. Apart from decoration the aim is to be able to stimulate his partner more effectively. Piercing can be dangerous if done carelessly. Important structures may be damaged and infection is a major risk. Some doctors will provide a piercing service, and this should reduce the risks.

Q MY HUSBAND IS ALWAYS TALKING ABOUT HOW HE WANTS TO WATCH ME MAKE LOVE TO OTHER MEN. HE USUALLY TALKS ABOUT THIS WHEN WE ARE MAKING LOVE AND I AM HAPPY TO GO ALONG WITH WHAT I'VE ALWAYS THOUGHT OF AS SIMPLY A FANTASY. BUT I HAVE HEARD OF SOME COUPLES WHO REALLY DO THIS AND NOW I AM WORRIED. THIS IS SOMETHING I DON'T WANT TO DO. WHAT ARE THE CHANCES OF MY HUSBAND'S FANTASY BECOMING A REALITY?

A Many men confess that they regularly fantasize about encouraging their regular partner to make love to one or more other men. In the fantasy, the arranged infidelity usually takes place in the husband's presence so that he can watch – and then make love to his partner after the other man has finished. Sometimes the female partner will be encouraged to make love to more than one man at once or to other women. This fantasy does not often turn into reality but it sometimes does. There are real dangers. First, there is the risk of infection. And secondly, there is the risk that the introduction of an additional partner will result in permanent damage being done to a long-standing relationship. You should explain to your husband that although you are happy to share his fantasy world, you will not allow his fantasy to become reality.

Q MY GIRLFRIEND SAYS SHE WANTS US TO MAKE LOVE IN PUBLIC. IS THIS NORMAL?

A Many people get a thrill from the risk of being discovered. Surprisingly large numbers of men and women have made love in parks, on trains, in planes, on boats and in lifts. The hazard of discovery can undoubtedly add excitement to a sexual relationship.

Q MY HUSBAND RECENTLY BROUGHT HOME A PORNOGRAPHIC MOVIE WHICH WE WATCHED TOGETHER. MUCH TO MY SURPRISE I FOUND IT SEXUALLY STIMULATING AND WHEN WE MADE LOVE AFTERWARDS IT WAS REALLY GOOD. I DIDN'T THINK THAT WOMEN FOUND BLUE MOVIES A TURN-ON. AM I ABNORMAL?

A No, you're not abnormal. Four out of five women are turned on by watching sexually explicit material. Some surveys have shown that women are more likely to be sexually stimulated by pornographic movies than men!

Q MY HUSBAND LIKES ME TO WEAR BLACK STOCKINGS WHEN WE MAKE LOVE. IS THIS FETISH DANGEROUS?

A A fetish is only really a fetish when it takes over. If your husband can enjoy sex without you wearing black stockings then he is merely telling you what turns him on. If he cannot get aroused at all unless you are wearing black stockings then he has developed a fetish that could get more and more out of control. Many men are turned on by particular types of clothes (black stockings are probably the commonest).

Q I HAVE TROUBLE PASSING URINE. IT TAKES A LONG TIME TO START AND THEN WHEN IT DOES

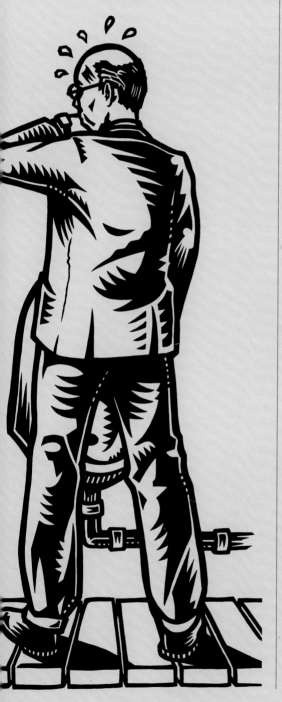

START THE STREAM IS VERY SLOW. DO YOU THINK I COULD HAVE AN INFECTION? I AM A 55-YEAR-OLD MALE.

A I think it is far more likely that you have an enlarged prostate gland – which is impeding the flow of urine from your bladder. A quick physical examination should enable your doctor to confirm the diagnosis. If you do have an enlarged prostate, then an operation to remove all or part of the enlarged gland should relieve your symptoms.

Q MY GIRLFRIEND ONLY ALLOWS ME TO MAKE LOVE TO HER WHILE SHE IS WEARING HER PANTIES. SHE SAYS THAT THIS MEANS THAT SHE IS STILL A VIRGIN. IS SHE RIGHT?

A Not if your penis enters her vagina. And if you ejaculate in or close to her vagina she can get pregnant.

Q MY HUSBAND LIKES TO TIE ME UP WHEN WE MAKE LOVE. HE IS CLEARLY TURNED ON BY IT. AND SO AM I. IS THIS DANGEROUS?

A Many couples add extra spice to their sex lives by tying one another up. Some women enjoy the feeling that they are being overpowered and forced to take part in sex acts about which they would otherwise feel guilty. Many men get a thrill from being tied up too. Remember, however, that bondage is not about hurting and it should be done with the consent of both partners. Make sure that your husband always ties knots that can be easily undone (by you if necessary). If your husband uses a gag make sure that you can remove it yourself if necessary. Don't let him tie anything around your neck, don't get into bondage after drinking alcohol and always arrange a code of some kind so that if you want to stop, you can communicate this to your husband.

Q MY GIRLFRIEND LIKES ME TO RIP HER CLOTHES OFF WHEN WE MAKE LOVE. I DON'T MIND BUT IS IT NORMAL?

A Lots of women like having their clothes torn off. But when you start make it clear what you are about to do and stop if she tells you to stop. Tearing her most expensive dress to shreds may prove expensive foreplay.

Q WHEN MY BOYFRIEND AND I STARTED TO LIVE TOGETHER WE HAD AN ACTIVE SEX LIFE

AND MADE LOVE AT LEAST TWICE A DAY. NOW WE HARDLY MAKE LOVE AT ALL. DO YOU THINK THIS MEANS HE IS BORED WITH ME?

A No. This is normal. A wise old man once told a young couple that if they put a penny into a jar every time they made love for the first six months of their marriage they would never empty the jar if they took a penny out every time they made love for the rest of their lives. Every young couple starting out together will claim that this is nonsense. But most couples who have been together for some time will confirm that he was right.

Q WHY DO MEN ONLY LIKE BIG BREASTS?

A Men are fascinated by breasts. But contrary to your suspicion they are fascinated by breasts of all shapes and sizes. Big ones, small ones, droopy ones, pert ones – all sizes and shapes have their own admirers.

Q I ALWAYS USED TO SHAVE MY LEGS BECAUSE I THOUGHT MEN LIKED SMOOTH LEGS BUT MY BOYFRIEND SAYS HE LIKES THEM LEFT UNSHAVED. WHICH DO MOST MEN PREFER?

A Two-thirds of men like women to shave their legs and a third prefer them to leave their legs unshaven and hairy.

Q DO MEN GO THROUGH A MENOPAUSE?

A Men don't have a hormonal change like women do but between the ages of forty and fifty most go through a period when they feel (and behave) strangely. They realize that time is running out, that much of what they are doing with their lives is irrelevant and that they are no longer young. They also worry about fading sexuality. All this frequently leads to a second adolescence, with an affair with a young mistress an occasional consequence.

Q WHAT CHANGES TAKE PLACE IN SEXUALITY AS WE GET OLDER?

A 1. Women's vaginas tend to be rather dry.
2. Men tend to have fewer erections and the

ones they get may not be quite as hard as they once were.
3. Sexual needs and desires diminish a little (though they don't disappear).
4. It takes a man longer to get an erection when he is older.
5. Premature ejaculation is uncommon among older men. They are usually able to maintain an erection for much longer before ejaculation takes place.
6. His orgasm will probably be slightly less explosive. There will be less semen.
7. It may take him longer than before to manage a second erection after making love.
8. She will take longer to get aroused and her vagina will take longer to become moistened.
9. Her vagina tends to expand less as she gets older, so it may seem tighter than it used to be. At the same time the vaginal walls will lose some of their grip.
10. Her orgasm will be less dramatic and she will be less likely to have multiple orgasms.

Q MY HUSBAND HAD A HEART ATTACK SIX MONTHS AGO. HIS DOCTOR SAYS WE CAN MAKE LOVE AGAIN. BUT WHICH POSITION WILL BE SAFEST FOR HIM?

A The woman on top positions may put less strain on him than man on top positions. Here are some simple rules.
1. Don't do anything that is painful.
2. If he is in pain then stop straight away.
3. Choose your positions carefully.
4. Don't let him drink alcohol or have a heavy meal before sex.

Q MY WIFE HAS TERRIBLE ARTHRITIS. BUT WE BOTH ENJOY MAKING LOVE. IS THERE ANYTHING WE CAN DO TO MAKE THINGS EASIER?

A Make sure that the room is warm. A warm bath beforehand may help too. Heat helps to make the joints more mobile.

Q MY PENIS IS VERY SMALL. HOW IMPORTANT IS SIZE TO A WOMAN?

A Only three per cent of women complain that their partner's penis is too small. It is what you do with it that really matters.

Q Is it normal for a happily married woman to enjoy flirting?
A Yes. Two out of three women enjoy flirting with men other than their regular partners, even though they have happy relationships.

Q What percentage of women use vibrators?
A Just under half of all women use vibrators.

Q My husband will not perform cunnilingus on me even though he expects me to perform oral sex on him. How can I persuade him that this is not fair.
A He's probably shy and anxious and needs encouragement. To start with ask him to kiss your vagina and then allow him to make his own progress. Make sure, however, that you wash thoroughly beforehand.

Q I recently found out that my husband spends his Sunday lunchtimes watching strip shows at a club. I was horrified. How many men do this?
A About a quarter of all men watch strip shows or live sex shows.

Q How common is it for a couple to have sex every day?
A Only about one in twenty steady couples have sex every day.

Q Are genital warts catching?
A Yes. The incidence is increasing. Genital warts are caused by a virus and transmitted by sexual contact. They need to be treated by a doctor. See page 106.

Q What is the difference between lust and love?
A You are in 'lust' when your feelings about someone are entirely physical. The stronger the physical attraction the greater the chances that it is lust. 'Love at first sight' usually means 'lust at first sight'. Love is wanting to be with someone, share things and experiences, look after them, protect them and hold them. Love is affection and friendship more than sex. You are in love when you realize that the person you are kissing is your best friend.

Q If a couple make love when the woman is pregnant is it possible for the penis to damage the baby?
A This is very unlikely. The average penis is neither big enough nor strong enough.

Q I am pregnant and my breasts are swollen and my nipples are huge. I feel embarrassed. Is my husband likely to find me repulsive in this condition?
A No. Many men find that pregnancy – and the changes that take place in a woman's body during it – makes a woman even more attractive, not less.

Q I've just had a baby. How can I get the tone back into my vaginal muscles? I want to be able to squeeze my husband as tightly as I could before the baby.
A There is a very simple routine that you can follow, outlined on page 75.

Q Can men get thrush?
A Yes. Most doctors treat the male partner if a woman has thrush because the infection can be passed backwards and forwards. Sometimes men have no symptoms even though they are carrying the infection. See page 107 for more information about thrush.

Q How many calories are burned up while making love?
A About 150 calories each. If you make love twice a week then, all other things being equal, in a year you will be about four pounds lighter.

Good Sex Index

Photographic Acknowledgements

The publishers would like to thank the following organizations
for their kind permission to reproduce the photographs in this book:
Bridgeman/Victor Lownes Collection/London 37;
Sally and Richard Greenhill 83 bottom; Hulton Deutsch/Bert Hardy 30;
The Hutchison Library 84; The Kobal Collection 24, /John Engstead 27;
Rex 109, /Sipa/Buguin/Sichov 28; Science Photo Library/Oscar Burriel/Latin Stock 89,
/Don Fawcett 90, /Professors P.M. Motta and J. Van Blerkom 11, /SIU 95;
Tony Stone Worldwide/Peter Correz 82, /Paul Dance, 25
/Ken Fisher 83 top; Zefa 31, 106.

Special Photography

Richard Truscott 2, 4, 7, 22, 32, 35, 59, 61,
63, 66, 71, 76, 81, 86, 87, 92, 99, 103,

Illustration

Kevin O'Keefe 97
Jared Gilbey 55, 56, 58
Patricia Ludlow 38 – 53 (all)

Line Artwork

Jared Gilbey 8, 9, 13, 15, 16, 18, 20,
67, 73, 75, 100, 101
Simon David 111 – 123 (all)

Art Direction Sarah Pollock
Design by Four Corners
Editor Sian Facer
Production Simon Shelmerdine
Picture Research Judy Todd